CORROSIVE REFORM:

FAILING HEALTH SYSTEMS IN EASTERN EUROPE

Carl Warren Afford

A joint publication by the International Labour Office
Socio-Economic Security Programme, Geneva
and Public Services International, Ferney-Voltaire

Cataloguing-in-publication data is available on request from INFORM, International Labour Office, CH-1211 Geneva 22, email INFORM@ilo.org

Afford, C.W.
Corrosive reform: failing health systems in Eastern Europe
Geneva, International Labour Office, 2003

Employment, conditions of employment, working conditions, wages, medical personnel, health service, Eastern Europe, 13.01.3

ISBN: 92-2-113705-8

ILO Cataloguing in Publication Data

Printed by the International Labour Office, Geneva, Switzerland

CONTENTS

Figures

Contents

Tables

ACKNOWLEDGEMENT

This Monograph is very much indebted to three reports prepared for the International Labour Organization (ILO) and Public Services International (PSI) "Failing Health Systems: Failing Health Workers in Eastern Europe", "Health Care in Central and Eastern Europe: Reform, Privatization and Employment in Four Countries" and "The Socio-Economic Status of Health Care Workers in the Russian Federation". Thanks are due therefore to the ILO InFocus Programme on Socio-Economic Security (IFP/SES); PSI; Charles Woolfson of the University of Glasgow; Andrew Watterson of the University of Sterling; and Matthias Beck of Glasgow Caledonian University; and to Natalia Stepantchikova, Liana Lakunina and Tatyana Tchetvernina of the Centre for Labour Market Studies, Institute of Economics, Russian Academy of Sciences.

As important, was the opportunity to apply the conceptual framework developed by IFP-SES for mapping and analysing socio-economic security within the health sphere and the work of IFP-SES team is acknowledged as are the very particular inputs of Guy Standing, Director and Ellen Rosskam, ILO IFP/SES, and Alan Leather of the PSI. There is also a debt of gratitude to all those PSI affiliates who were instrumental in replying to ILO/PSI survey and in answering follow up questions. The Workshop on "Health Care Privatization: Workers' Insecurities in Eastern Europe" convened by ILO/PSI in Geneva, 2001 allowed some of the initial thinking in this analysis to be tested and provided information from national trade union leaders. Gratitude is due to the organizers of the meeting and all its participants. The ideas of the "Joint Meeting on the Social Dialogue in Health Services: Institutions, Capacity and Effectiveness" and its conclusions were also highly valued. The work of the health for all database of WHO Regional Office for Europe and of the European Observatory on Health Care Systems and the Health Care Systems in Transition series is acknowledged with gratitude. Special thanks are extended to all those who contributed ideas, comments or reviews including (in alphabetical order) Adrian Birca, Romanian Trade Union Federation SANITAS; Ainna Fawcett-Henesy, WHO Regional Office for Europe; Thomas E. Novotny, Institute of Global Health, University of California; Bill Ratteree and Christiane Wiskow, Health Services, Sectoral Activities Department, ILO; Alan Rowe, Naken Saaliev, Health Trade Union of Kyrgyzstan; Ulle Schmidt, Chair, Federation of Estonian Health Care Professionals Unions; Mariya Telishevska, Associate Professor, Lviv State Medical University, Jiří Schlanger and Jana Vesela, Trade Union of the Health Service and Social Care of the Czech Republic. Thanks also to Julie Lim who has provided administrative support.

BACKGROUND

1

This Monograph takes forward the analysis of three International Labour Organization (ILO) and Public Services International (PSI) reports on the socio-economic security of health care workers in Central and Eastern Europe (CEE) and the Commonwealth of Independent States (CIS). They and the very considerable research that preceded them have been invaluable in shaping this current work.

No one industry or sector is quite like any other, and those involved in health policy-making, and the planning, finance and delivery of health care argue that health is a unique commodity. Certainly, there are particular values and notions of rights attached to it and health economics describes the market for health as different, or "special" (ILO, 2000a). The health care sector however is also, a very significant force in terms of employment. Health care systems account for hundreds of thousands of jobs across Europe and those human resources account for a major part of the costs of health care systems. A great deal of research and negotiation has been focused on both the health and the employment dimensions of the sector and the intersection of the two. Much of that work underpins this and other recent studies. It draws for example on ILO Conventions, particularly the Nursing Personnel Convention, 1977 (No. 149) and Recommendation, 1977 (No. 157), as well as on relevant agreements from the health sphere such as the Ljubljana Charter, which was agreed by the 1996 WHO Regional Office for Europe Conference and established guidance on developing and reforming the health care systems of Europe.

The ILO Joint Committee for Health Services has also generated a number of meetings, negotiations and studies over the past decade, which has informed this work. Amongst them was the ILO/PSI Workshop on Employment and Labour Practices in Health Care in CEE, in Prague in 1997. It gave rise to a significant background paper [1] and moved forward the agenda set out by the Committee in 1992, undertaking to "create awareness of the need for social dialogue, to develop the means to implement it, and to establish the importance of working conditions in the context of improving the quality of health care delivery" (ILO, 1998).

---

[1] The study was undertaken in 1995/96, and published as an ILO sectoral working paper (Healy and Humphries, 1997).

Corrosive reform: Failing health systems in Eastern Europe

The 1998 ILO sectoral meeting on "Terms of Employment and Working Conditions in Health Sector Reforms" advanced this process further recommending "in the health sector reform process, policies should be developed for social dialogue since the best reforms are developed through such dialogue". The report prepared for the meeting examined global trends in the sector and was supplemented by the subsequent 1998 report produced for the 1999 Almaty Conference on "Employment and Working Conditions in the Health Sector of Central Asian Countries". Its aim was to "provide assistance through regional workshops with the aim of making improvements to both the health services themselves and the employment conditions of health workers". It explored both the health and employment interface and the implications of privatization for workers, (an emerging issue at that time). These meetings and reports, and the more recent 2002 Joint Meeting on Social Dialogue in the Health Services, have highlighted the employment and security challenges faced by health workers and the need to engage with them in developing health system reforms in order to "facilitate the implementation of new, improved approaches to health services" (ILO, 2002b).

The Workshop on "Health Care Privatization: Workers' Insecurities in Eastern Europe', convened by ILO/PSI in Geneva, 2001, was particularly relevant. It prompted the development of the three background papers and ultimately this study itself and provided significant (ILO/PSI) survey data, which has illuminated the extent of the insecurity of health sector workers. Perhaps as importantly it was an opportunity to apply the conceptual framework developed by the ILO InFocus Programme on Socio-Economic Security (IFP/SES) for mapping and analysing socio-economic security within the health sphere. The framework identifies seven dimensions of socio-economic security that together capture the totality of workers' experiences of security and insecurity. It is robust enough to encapsulate the concerns of health workers and has guided this analysis. The seven dimensions are:

- labour market security: adequate employment opportunities, through state-guaranteed full employment, or at least high levels of employment ensured by macro-economic policy;

- employment security: protection against arbitrary dismissal, regulations on hiring and firing, imposition of costs on employers, etc.;

- job security: a niche designated as an occupation of "career", plus tolerance of demarcation practices, barriers to skill dilution, craft boundaries, job qualifications, restrictive practices, craft unions, etc.;

- skill reproduction security: widespread opportunities to gain and retain skills, through apprenticeships, employment training, etc.;

- work security: protection against accidents and illness at work, through safety and health regulations, limits on working time, unsociable hours, night work for women, etc.;

- representation security: protection of a collective voice in the labour market, through independent trade unions and employer associations incorporated economically and politically into the state, with the right to strike, etc.;

- income security: protection of income through minimum wage, wage indexation, comprehensive social security, progressive taxation, etc.

Finally, this Monograph owes a debt of gratitude to the authors of the "Draft Report to the Joint Meeting on the Social Dialogue in Health Services: Institutions, Capacity and Effectiveness" who provide enormous insights into current thinking in this field.

Recent research

The ILO IFP-SES and PSI undertook a major research project in 2000-2001 on health workers' security and commissioned two studies in the area. These, together with a report on the Russian health care system and the views of PSI affiliates formed the basis of discussions at the ILO/PSI Geneva workshop on privatization in health care in 2001 (see above). The three reports "Failing Health Systems: Failing Health Workers in Eastern Europe" (Afford, 2001), "Health Care in Central and Eastern Europe: Reform, Privatization and Employment in Four Countries" (ILO, 2001) and "The Socio-Economic Status of Health Care Workers in the Russian Federation" (Stepantchikova et al., 2001) all fed into this work.

The study, "Failing Health Systems: Failing Health Workers", used empirical evidence in an attempt to quantify and assess the impact of a decade of reforms on health sector staff in CEE and CIS. The study drew heavily on data provided by fifteen PSI affiliates who completed the Basic Security Survey (ILO/PSI Survey)[2] for the years 1990-1999, specifically Armenia, Belarus, Bulgaria, Croatia, Czech Republic, Kyrgyzstan, Georgia, Latvia, Lithuania, the Republic of Moldova, Poland, Romania, the Russian Federation, Slovakia, and Ukraine. The aim of the research was to assess the insecurities of health workers in light of the seven socio-economic security dimensions as defined by IFP-SES. The socio-economic position of the region at large and the sweeping health sector reforms that had taken place during the decade long reference period were

---

[2] This questionnaire was developed by IFP-SES and PSI and was originally sent to 35-PSI trade union affiliates across the region.

also examined, providing some background to the study and an explanation of the context in which the technical evidence was gathered.

The second, simultaneous study examined in-depth, four countries seen to be representative of the region; the Czech Republic, Lithuania, Romania, and Ukraine. It sought to "gauge how restructuring has affected the working conditions of individual health care workers" by exploring workers' experiences linked to working hours, physical conditions, changes in tasks performed, union representation and income (including non-payment of wages). The study applied a "multi-dimensional" approach, combining interviews and surveys of management, government representatives, union officials and worker representatives as well as individual employees[3]. A strategic sample of institutions regarded as "typical of the sector"[4] was investigated in each of the four countries, with the co-operation of trade union representatives and, wherever possible, hospital management[5]. The results of the survey (in graphic form) identify common themes in the working lives of health care workers and the differences between staff in the four countries.

Finally, a third component was commissioned by IFP/SES to investigate evidence on the health care sector in the Russian Federation. It aimed to assess the socio-economic situation of the country's health care workers and to set that in the wider context of the problems besetting the health care sector. The report examined the working conditions, income and skill security of staff in detail and examined the gap between official data and workers' experience[6]. Evidence was drawn from official documents and statistics provided by the Ministry of Health Care and the National Statistics Committee and interviewed health care staff and their representatives, illustrating vividly the challenges that Russian workers face.

In addition to the research and reports provided through the ILO IFP-SES/PSI research project, this analysis draws extensively on the employment policy and health systems literature, and supplementary materials, to provide a wider and deeper understanding of the situation in the health sector across CEE and CIS. These reports and articles are cited throughout the text that follows.

---

[3] In total the authors received 2,215 individual responses to the questionnaire from health care workers, 466 from the Czech Republic, 834 from Lithuania, 735 from Ukraine, and 180 from Romania.

[4] The institutions sampled included polyclinics, and a secondary care hospital or a specialist tertiary institution. See report for full details and weighting.

[5] Although union support was provided, both union and non-union staff were surveyed.

[6] The authors explicitly preface their analysis with the recognition that "official statistics do not provide complete information, especially on issues of employment in the health care sector". The authors also point out that "information about the private sector (and, with few exceptions, about the departmental medical institutions) is not available".

Scope and aim

The aim of this research has been to provide an overview of the immense changes that have taken place in the health systems of CEE and CIS over the past 12 years and to examine the impact of these changes on the health care workers of the region. It has also been to place the transformations in health in the context of the wider economy so that workers' experience of change can be properly understood.

Health care reforms have been implemented in all the countries of CEE and CIS and in almost all cases have brought about wide-ranging changes in how care is funded, organized and delivered to the public at large. This in turn has transformed the demands made on the workers involved in providing that care. There are two particularly relevant strands of analysis. The first sets out the employment perspective. It involves detailed studies, carried out for the ILO and PSI and focuses on the effects of reforms and budget constraints on medical and general health sector staff. The second focuses on health systems literature and is primarily concerned with the efficient allocation of scarce resources, the values ascribed to health care provision and the user-provider (-payer) relationship.

These two strands of analysis are brought together here in order to understand the contextual and motivating factors that have led countries to choose particular reforms and to explore their implications for the staff affected. It aims therefore to marry an understanding of the policy imperatives of health system reforms with empirical survey findings on employment, thereby examining the correlation between reforming organizational structures and workers' security. The purpose of this is to provide the evidence and insights necessary for national and international actors to enhance the security of the health sector workforce and so maximize the chances of health care reforms being effective. A number of concrete recommendations have been generated and it is hoped that these, as well as the overall analysis will contribute to the work of the ILO in its attempts to secure "Decent Work for All".

The piece of work should be seen as a continuation of previous studies on the challenges facing health workers in Eastern Europe and as part of ongoing efforts to convince decision-makers that social dialogue is both the best means of addressing working conditions and a precursor to improving the quality of health care.

A caveat

This Monograph seeks to provide a realistic picture of the situation in CEE and CIS, but it is essential that the size and diversity of the region is appreciated. There can be no single context where 28 countries are concerned. Clearly the communist systems in place before transition and the particular dominance of the Soviet Union meant an enormous amount that was shared, not least the structure and approach to health care provision which was overwhelmingly influenced by the Semashko model. Nonetheless, the region is composed of different national and ethnic groups speaking different languages and with very different historical and cultural heritages, economic and mineral resources. The transition process has seen many groups strive for autonomy and/or nationhood and a re-emergence of their distinct traditions.

This caveat is important as it effects how health is perceived and valued. Decisions about how to organize health systems or structure payments for health care will also be influenced by each country's historical experiences and national culture (Afford, 2001). It goes without saying that the influences on the Czech Republic or Hungary with their pre-communist experiences of social insurance will differ from those that hold sway in central Asian countries which will differ in turn from the factors that are important to the constituent parts of the former Yugoslavia. Indeed just as there are different expectations and cultural legacies, there are varying degrees of linkage with Western Europe. The German government has historic ties with Slovenia and Croatia, the Finnish government with the Baltic States and the Russian Federation; these too will affect approaches to reform. Similarly, the EU will be increasingly important in shaping elements of health and employment policy, if only in the more affluent countries of CEE.

The way workers are regarded and treated will also depend on factors that vary across the region. The role allowed for trade unions and attitudes to solidarity will be shaped by national politics, recent history and perhaps a need to draw a line under what has gone before. Some countries may seek to establish a new identity by rejecting the past and asserting their membership in market economies. Some may pursue credibility with the west by adopting policies favoured by international financial institutions.

All generalizations about socio-economic security must therefore be understood in light of these caveats, and not as a denial of the differences between the countries of the region.

CONTEXT

2

The human impact of transition

Eastern Europe is not an amorphous mass. It is an immensely diverse region. Yet every single country in it has suffered enormously going through "transition". The collapse of the economies of CEE and CIS in the early 1990s is common knowledge. The extent of that collapse and the severity of its impact on the workers of the region are however more difficult to comprehend. Stagflation, restructuring and burgeoning unemployment contributed to a devastating rise in poverty, growing disparities between rich and poor and falling life expectancy. By the end of the 1990s only Poland, Hungary and Slovakia had achieved or almost achieved their 1989 level of GDP (Dunford and Smith, 2000). Employment across the region declined by some 9 per cent for men and by 13 per cent for women between 1989 and 1996. Behind these statistics were 11.7 million people who lost their jobs, 7.2 million of them women (ILO, 1997). The reduction in labour force participation was even more marked and even harder to grasp, with vast numbers of workers "disappearing". Comparing changes in employment and unemployment (table 1) demonstrates how many of the Czech, Hungarian and Lithuanian workers who lost their jobs in the early 1990s became non-participants in the labour market. They may have retired early or been pushed into early retirement. Many will have engaged in some precarious informal activity. Whatever the explanation they dropped out of the formal economy and were no longer captured by employment and unemployment statistics. This pattern was repeated again and again. While not all those withdrawing or "being withdrawn" from the labour market necessarily fall into poverty, the evidence of increased ill health, premature death, homelessness, destitution, emigration, forced work in the sex industry and the abandonment of children speak volumes about the extent of impoverishment in the region.

For many, transition translated to a collapse in life expectancy. Middle-aged men in particular died prematurely and in vast numbers. The precise causes are debated but the immense stress associated with job losses and poverty, falling nutritional status and problematic coping mechanisms including misuse of alcohol and tobacco have all contributed to increased accidents, violence and excess morbidity and mortality. Rising rates of tuberculosis (TB) which are associated with worsening living conditions, the appearance of multi-drug resistant TB and the emergence and re-emergence of sexually transmitted infections, including the spread of AIDS, have all taken a toll, particularly in parts of the former Soviet Union (Chenet *et al.*, 1996; Stepantchikova *et al.*, 2001). While the worst of the initial reaction has passed and life expectancy has started to recover, the stressors and dislocation that prompted damaging behaviours and contributed to the appalling health outcomes are still in place.

Table 1. Employment and unemployment changes in CEE, 1990–1996 (per cent change)

Country	Change in employment	Change in unemployment	Ratio
Slovakia	-12.07	12.0	0.99
Poland	-13.58	11.3	0.83
Russian Federation (data 1991-96)	-10.63	8.3	0.78
Estonia (data 1990-94)	-10.75	7.9	0.73
Bulgaria	-19.64	11.5	0.58
Latvia (data 1992-96)	-13.17	6.2	0.47
Czech Republic	-6.36	2.8	0.44
Lithuania (data 1991-96)	-12.57	5.2	0.41
Hungary	-26.75	8.9	0.33

Note: Figures are expressed as a per cent change from the initial level relative to the initial labour force. A ratio of 1.00 (assuming no change in the working-age population) means every worker who lost a job entered formal unemployment. A ratio below 1.00 indicates workers losing jobs and disappearing from the labour market.

Source: Elaborated from ILO in Work, Employment and Transition (Rainnie, Smith and Swain, 1996. 1997).

The position of health care workers in CEE and CIS over the last dozen years must be seen in this context. Like everyone else they have experienced the impact of economic collapse, the pressures on the public sector and the uncertainties of restructuring. On top of this they have faced the strains of tending to a population in distress. They treat the men who die young in the face of social upheaval and the children with diseases of poverty. In the midst of this they must cope as best they can with scarce resources and huge insecurity.

Economic and employment impacts; devastating transitions

It was inevitable that there should be huge disruption across the region as the mutually dependent communist systems were replaced with competing market economies. At the very least the break up of the former Soviet Union into 16 separate countries was bound to cause chaos. The whole Soviet economy had been managed as a single entity with production allocated between Republics. Tractors made in Minsk depended on the transfer of parts from the Baltic, parts which from 1991 could only be imported from a different country with a different currency. Pharmaceuticals production was arranged in the same way, to benefit the whole USSR, but is now divided between independent countries.

Soviet experiments with monoculture in agricultural production and its predilection for what were virtually "company" towns also exacerbated the problems of independence with new nations left to deal with the environmental and social legacy of past patterns of production. It also meant an end to subsidies between Republics, which had significant implications for the poorest (ILO, 2000a). Although it would be true to say that the Soviet Union never achieved total equity of allocation of resources despite its widespread use of norms, it did allow for transfers to central Asia or other areas experiencing difficulties. This has now ceased completely. Indeed it was not just the former Soviet Union, which was faced with a loss of traditional markets and the breakdown of transfers between regions. Trade across the whole of the Eastern bloc was profoundly affected and there was an unravelling of industrial production and the markets of what were the COMECON countries. This contributed to job losses, inflation induced impoverishment and social suffering.

Workers right across the region and in all sectors, not just health, were particularly ill prepared to cope with labour market insecurity because of the way employment was organized and the "cradle to grave" services to which they had been accustomed. This is not to suggest that the people of CEE and CIS did not exercise considerable initiative and entrepreneurial flair in supplementing their income and enriching their lifestyles, but it was the *statal* system, which guaranteed all their physiological needs. All the centrally planned economies were premised on full (compulsory) employment with labour intensive rather than capital-intensive models meeting social objectives. A shift away from cash based payments which "commodified" labour had been engineered in favour of an approach dependent on a high level of social transfers in-kind, or rather, in the form of services. This meant that individuals were paid a wage that was to provide for a single adult rather than a family, and that while all adults were expected to work, family (as opposed to "individual") needs were largely met through social transfers and vià the transmission belt of enterprise, party and trade unions (Standing, 1996). Almost all women worked, the disabled worked, even pensioners worked albeit that pay rates were low and women were concentrated in lower paid jobs. The enterprise and/or the state provided subsidized housing, childcare, health services and leisure facilities. The delivery of social transfers was so intimately connected with work, that there were scarcely any benefit systems designed to operate independently of the employment sphere. What is more, the unemployed were widely regarded as parasitic or criminal. People participated in the labour market not in a western European sense for their pay, but for the combination of benefits and entitlements that came with work. Employment was very much the key to membership of the system. The impact of the collapse of socialist labour markets and the subsequent economic reforms was therefore all the more profound.

The economic advisers, the international community and above all international financial institutions who sought to guide transition fostered a particular approach to market reforms, an approach which was often enthusiastically taken up by post-communist governments. The presumption underpinning the economic policy they advocated was that price liberalization would be a key motor for change. It was to create market relations, prompt the tightening of fiscal policy and depress demand and public spending. These coupled with privatization were to force enterprises to pursue efficiency. Enterprises were expected to respond by reforming employment and revitalizing production thus delivering economic regeneration. Price liberalization was advocated as a first step, which would lead on via stabilization and privatization to restructuring.

This sequencing of reforms proved wholly inappropriate (Standing, 1997). Price liberalization in what were highly monopolistic economies (and in advance of restructuring) led to spiralling inflation, the indebtedness of enterprises and a widespread collapse in production and labour markets. While manufacturing industries and utilities were the most obvious focus of market reforms and were the initial targets for privatization, the public sector was also profoundly affected. Governments were under enormous pressure to reduce budget deficits and in the face of falling production and dwindling tax revenues[7] they responded (as prompted) by cutting public expenditure and investment in the social infrastructure, in what has been termed "state desertion". The effects of liberalization combined with these draconian attempts at stabilization caused havoc in societies, which did not have social security systems able to deal with mass unemployment. The expectation that it would do otherwise was optimistic if not foolhardy.

In some respects the international agencies and financial institutions that advised on the restructuring of Eastern Europe had tacitly recognized the devastation that would be wreaked by reducing job numbers in that they advocated the establishment of social support systems as a adjunct to "shock therapies" (Standing, 2002). Their commitment to the market model of transition however, meant this support was envisaged as a safety net only. The IMF and World Bank in particular made minimizing the cost of such social provision a key objective, and through conditions attached to lending programmes, insisted on liberal and neo-liberal approaches to social and employment policy that inserted fundamental inadequacies into the systems developed[8]. The benefits put in place have therefore tended to be selective and to depend on means testing in order to "target" those deemed worthy of support. This has been highly problematic because the lack of established infrastructure for delivering benefits, the legacy of stigmatization and hostility to those not in work and the sheer unfamiliarity of people with the paraphernalia of benefit systems have made it particularly hard for people in need to secure their entitlements.

---

[7] Tax revenues fell not only as a consequence of the collapse of manufacturing but also because of wide spread tax avoidance, which is discussed in more detail below.

[8] Role of international financial institutions (IFIs) in Gowan (1995) and Wedle (2000), cited by Rainnie et al., 2002.

The inadequacies of the benefit system in many CEE and CIS countries are compounded by the link that national policy-makers have been encouraged to make between benefit levels and the minimum wage. Governments have knowingly allowed the minimum wage to fall well below subsistence levels, often under direct pressure from international agencies, most specifically the IMF. Bulgaria, Kyrgyzstan and the Russian Federation for example all have a minimum wage which remains resolutely below the official poverty line even when this has been revised downwards with some vigour and is less than is needed for basic survival (Standing, 1996). As Standing has demonstrated the minimum wage then becomes a tool of destitution rather than a guarantee of security. Indeed Standing and other commentators have also suggested that targeting selective benefits is expensive and ultimately a waste of funds; that it tends to give bureaucrats arbitrary and oppressive powers to determine who is or is not part of the deserving poor; and that, perversely, it discourages labour mobility or an appropriate mixing of formal and informal employment (Standing, 2002). Certainly in CEE and CIS it has contributed to the creation of a marginalized underclass and a very real threat that anyone losing their job will become trapped in a cycle of poverty and exclusion [9].

The "social safety net" promoted by the international community may have proved woefully inadequate and led to deprivation and poverty, in large part because of the flaws designed in to the system as a result of neo-liberal beliefs. However, there are additional and very substantial problems that stem from the crumbling of social transfers.

Transfers were traditionally transmitted via party, enterprises and trade unions and included significant amounts of in-kind benefits (see above). Many enterprises cut back on the provision of non-monetary benefits and closed down services during "stabilization" because they could no longer afford to maintain childcare, health and leisure facilities. Some compensated staff with cash remuneration although inevitably the replacement value of the monetary payments was less that it cost to purchase equivalent services in the new market place and inflation rapidly devalued the compensation package. Others managed to keep services going but consistently under invested in facilities reducing the value of provision. In theory, this need not have lead to workers losing out. Transfers in the form of employers' insurance contributions (as well as employees' contributions) and enterprise taxes should have replaced transfers in-kind and funded adequate bundles of benefits. However, just as the state system

---

[9] Some commentators claim that the informal economy and household survival strategies protect non-participants in the labour market and that formal employment and benefits are of diminishing importance (see Smith, Chapter 12 in *Work, Employment and Transition*). Clarke demonstrates (in the same volume Chapter 10) that although households do combine income sources to survive, marginal, private and subsistence activities alone cannot provide adequate security. Social transfers and declared, formal income remain hugely important, albeit that they are often supplemented with additional, sometimes informal income sources.

was called upon to fill the social benefit gap for those in work and to provide for the unemployed the amount of revenue collected plummeted.

Enterprises responded to the growing call for cash transfers to the state by seeking to evade the payment of insurance contributions and taxes. They routinely under declared revenues and, what is worse began to "casualize" labour, removing workers from "the books" and treating them as self-employed sub-contractors, since the nominally self-employed do not trigger the same insurance contributions. Staff colluded with this because of pressures from employers and because they had little confidence that the system would be able to deliver their entitlement to benefits in the future. It made sense therefore for them to opt for short-term cash payments instead of deferred entitlement (Standing, 1997). Irregular forms of employment and remuneration were also encouraged by the perverse incentives created by many tax-based incomes policies. These policies were promoted by international agencies and severely penalised enterprises for allowing average wage bills to rise. While this might have kept wages at levels that were attractive to international investors, it also prompted a shift from money wages into tax-free benefits [10], cash-in-hand and under-the-table payments that further reduced the formal revenue base and the level of social transfers (Standing, 1996). In the absence of adequate transfers local government declined to take on the service provision role vacated by so many enterprises, thus leading to shortfalls in services.

A final striking feature of the transformation of the centrally planned economies has been the recasting of the relationships between employers, management, employees and trade unions. Generalizations about an entire region obviously have their limitations but it is fair to say that in the communist era government was the all but universal owner-employer while unions (with a few notable exceptions) worked with government to promote productivity and as transmission belts for benefits. The labour process was based, in formal terms, on top down control but it consistently failed to achieve efficient coordination [11]. Instead there was unevenness of work and technology and considerable space for individual influence and negotiation. It is clear that workers were heavily dependent on the enterprise, and they may often have been alienated from their work and dominated by management as some commentators suggest. However, the notion that despotic and arbitrary factory regimes used piece rates and norms beyond the workers' control to impose oppressive discipline is less compelling when the actual powerlessness of supervisors to secure supplies or influence

---

[10]   A minority of enterprises, often the more successful and autarchic, have bucked the trend of replacing in-kind benefits with "monetarized" remuneration. They have maintained and enhanced enterprise-based service provision as a more tax efficient way of remunerating workers. This reduces transfers to the state as surely as casualizing labour and also polarizes the position of workers, increasing inequity.

[11]   The analysis of communist, and particularly Soviet, labour relations by Bahro, Burawoy, Mandel, Stark and others is described in more detail by Rainnie *et al.* (2002), pp.13–18.

---

how work was done is acknowledged. Rainnie, Smith and Swain suggest there was a feeling of mutual interest between managers and workers with alliances established to achieve basic production norms in the face of the "shortage economy".

The situation might more properly be described, as a community of "mutual disinterest" with managers and workers colluding with each other to secure a quite life and avoid the "scapegoating" that would follow overt failure to perform. Whatever the exact position in the various parts of the region, transition has transformed this style of "industrial relations". There has been increasing differentiation between employers and employees, between management and workers, and between employees of the private and public sector. It is no longer the case that all employees are employees of the state and workers have to adjust to a transformed labour market and to the new power of employers to "hire and fire". This in turn implies a new role for the trade union movement (Thirkell and Vickerstaff, 2002). Given that unions were so closely identified with the state and achieving "management" objectives it is striking that many played a part in the crises which led to change (albeit that some of these were new, independent unions). Initially many supported reform strategies; helping to negotiate new labour codes and some went on to be involved as social partners in tripartite initiatives. However, as the initial threats to post-transition economies have waned and "the hegemony of the neo-liberal model of economic reform remains unchallenged ... the scope for unions to extract employment and social policy concessions is largely undermined" (Thirkell and Vickerstaff, 2002, p. 68). Many governments under pressure to reduce wage costs and entitlements and in an effort to attract multi-national companies, are ever more reluctant to engage with unions, while international investors are often hostile to them and chose not to formally involve them in consultation processes. Unions are confronting new challenges often with a lack of resources and with falling income, and at times they struggle to overcome a legacy of distrust amongst members, some of whom perceive unions as increasingly powerless or even irrelevant (Stepantchikova *et al.*, 2001). Unions are often increasingly marginalized even though workers clearly need voice representation as much, if not more, than ever.

The international community, its financial institutions, the IMF, World Bank and investors, must all bear considerable responsibility for advocating an approach to economic transformation which exposed the people of CEE to such extremes of dislocation. Vast numbers were made unemployed, and even more were discouraged from participating in or forced out of the formal labour market. The sequencing of reforms and restructuring created a much greater need for the state to provide a "social safety net" than had ever been the case before, at precisely the time that revenues and social transfers were collapsing and governments were facing the most intense international pressures to cut public expenditure. Benefits systems have singularly failed to cope. Workers have also seen an entirely new set of industrial relations emerge while often the newly separated government and employers turn their back on trade unions. Those in work have no guarantees of adequate representation while those without work are voiceless. People welcomed the fall of communism and the opportunities market mechanisms were seen to represent, but the price they have paid during transition has been immense.

The impact of transition on the health sector

Change in the health sector must be seen both in the context of the wider economy and in light of its historical position in communist societies. The health sector before transition was regarded as "unproductive" and it was valued less than manufacturing or trade. Nonetheless, health services were regarded as a benefit that all workers were entitled to and as a cornerstone of efforts to produce the "next generation" of healthy workers. Staff may have been undervalued and relatively poorly paid [12] but the provision of care, particularly curative, occupational and rehabilitative health services, was an important component of the package of social transfers provided to workers. Provision was extensive, labour rather than capital intensive [13] and funded from global, tax-based budgets. It was normally organized in line with the Soviet Semashko model [14] and combined mainstream health service structures with parallel health systems linked to a range of Ministries and often to individual enterprises, which allowed workers to obtain health care in and through the work place [15]. There was a heavy reliance on centrally determined norms (of beds to head of population, and physicians and nurses to beds) with a quota of hospitals (in-patient care) and polyclinics (primary and specialist ambulatory care) per neighbourhood, district and region with tertiary, specialist hospitals concentrated at the apex of the system. Primary care was relatively undeveloped with a range of health posts and polyclinics offering first contact care but little in terms of health promotion and with only a limited capacity to refer upwards to secondary care and almost no gatekeeping function. Typically facility budgets were increased on the basis of historical incrementalism and in line with numbers of beds, staff and patient stays or visits. This created few incentives for efficiency or patient turnover and helped to sustain high staffing levels (Saltman and Figueras, 1997). This did not attract the attention of governments because health

---

[12] The low pay in health care may explain (or be explained by) the fact that the majority of staff including doctors were female, despite which men held the most senior medical positions.

[13] The numbers of physician and nurses per 1'000 population were high relative to norms in EU member states (for more details see Afford {2001} but total health sector employment was not as widely at odds with western European figures as is sometimes believed (see Section 3).

[14] There were exceptions, notably self-management in Yugoslavia, but the model was otherwise widespread (and was of course applied without exception in the Soviet republics).

[15] There were exceptions, notably self-management in Yugoslavia, but the model was otherwise widespread (and was of course applied without exception in the Soviet republics).

service unit costs were relatively cheap and because before transition public sector support to health services was unquestioned.

When the economies of CEE and CIS collapsed however, governments did little if anything to protect the value of their spending on health and some (perhaps in response to international pressure to reduce public expenditure) even cut the percentage of GDP devoted to health care (fig. 1). Data is incomplete but a comparison of spending in some European Union and transition countries gives a sense of the differences in norms. It does not however, reflect the relative value of the respective investment in health care or convey the tiny dollar sums per person being spent in most CEE and CIS countries. The assault on health spending was extreme, particularly in the face of price liberalization and stagflation, and it was translated into a chronic lack of public funds for investment and health sector pay.

Under investment in facilities and technology was not a new thing. Health sector conditions had been indifferent in much of the former Soviet Union and CEE and the focus on providing a high volume of beds (which was a misguided attempt to ensure sufficient capacity to respond to epidemics) consumed resources that might have otherwise been more effectively targeted. Nor was there a serious understanding of, or commitment to, quality services that would respond to individual patients' needs [16]. Health sector infrastructure was simply not a priority before transition. However, since transition there has been a further and often stark decline in conditions and a startling increase in inequity between regions. Low and falling health expenditures at a time when price liberalization sent the cost of medical supplies and pharmaceuticals soaring have created real and sometimes-insurmountable difficulties in meeting even the most basic health needs. In the early 1990s many health authorities found it impossible to maintain the fabric of hospitals and clinics. Hospital equipment suffered too and became increasingly outmoded or even obsolete. There were also insufficient resources to purchase the basics like bandages and syringes. Increasingly patients were expected to pay out-of-pocket for the consumables required to provide day-to-day care and there was a proliferation of under-the-table payments [17]. These inevitably created barriers to access to care undermining the principles of solidarity and equity, which underpin public health provision. These problems persist across much of the region and although there are exceptions with donor programmes making significant contributions to some institutions and others (often the formerly closed or elite hospitals) investing in facilities and equipment, conditions overall are still widely held to be inadequate and to contribute to poor staff morale (McKee and Healy, 2002).

---

[16] This is a comment on responsiveness to users and not on the technical quality of health services.

[17] It was commonplace in communist systems for an extensive informal economy to run in parallel with the formal economy. Health was not exempt and "gratitude payments" were widespread. The need for inpatients to purchase medical supplies and even food was new however.

Of course staff morale has also been undermined by significant erosion in the value of health sector pay. Even allowing for relatively low salary levels before transition, comparisons with other sectors and with national average pay provide little comfort for nurses, auxiliaries and administrators and not much more reassurance for doctors. For many health workers wages have been severely devalued and in some cases continue to fall behind the national average. In the immediate aftermath of transition health sector staff were often paid late, sometimes as much as three months in arrears, and although in most countries this is increasingly rare there are still instances of delayed payment and of the use of administrative leave. This has exacerbated the culture of gratitude payments and of parallel economic activity that existed before transition and there is evidence that an enormous amount of health expenditure is private, out-of-pocket and unregulated [18], although this does not imply that a large proportion of any individual's pay is "informal". Under-the-table payments may be problematic in terms of ensuring access to health care services but they also have serious implications for staff security. Informal pay is by definition difficult to measure or to regulate and is not amenable to distribution in line with transparent or agreed objectives. Occupational groups with direct contact with patients will inevitably have greater opportunities to supplement their income and the most powerful, i.e. doctors will be far better placed to control system resources and so to command gratuities. Administrative staff, auxiliaries and cleaners are likely to have the lowest pay and the least access to supplementary sources of income exacerbating inequities.

---

[18] Household expenditure surveys for Bulgaria suggest that about half of health sector revenue is from informal sources while the World Bank suggests that in Moldova only a fraction of costs are covered by the government (cited in Afford, 2001).

Figure 1.   Total health expenditure as percentage of GDP, 1990–2000 [19]

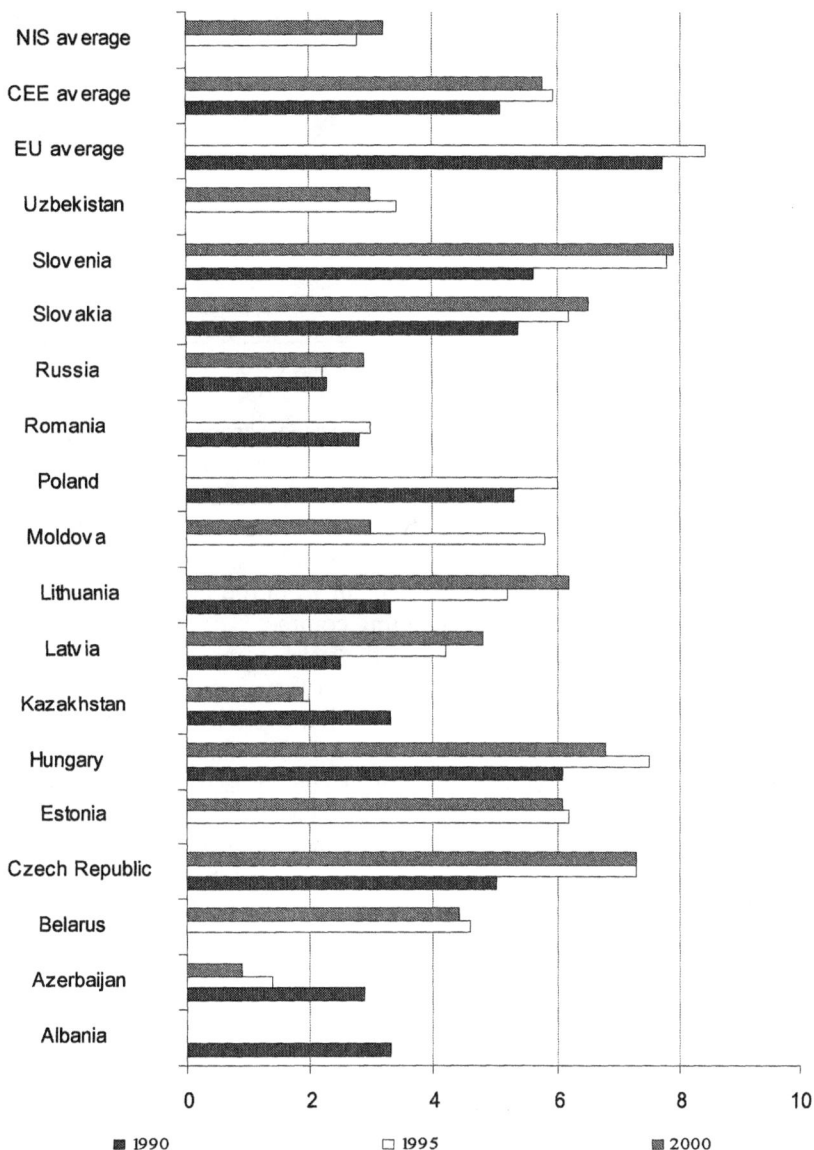

| | 1990 | 1995 | 2000 |

Source: WHO HFA (2002).

[19] The WHO Health for All Database gives averages for newly independent states (NIS) rather than the Commonwealth of Independent States (CIS), which is used here and does not include the Baltic States. CIS averages are not readily available but NIS data are offered as an indication of at least some regional trends.

Corrosive reform: Failing health systems of Eastern Europe

Table 2. Total expenditure on health as a percentage of GDP in selected CEE, NIS and western European countries, (1998)

Germany	10.7
France	9.6
European Union average	8.5
Czech Republic	7.2
United Kingdom	6.8
Central and Eastern European average	5.3
Lithuania	5.1
Ukraine	3.5
Romania	2.6

Source: Elaborated from WHO (1998) in Draft to the ILO–PSI 2001.

While pay continues to be a thorny issue across CEE and CIS, there have not been wholesale cuts in jobs, nor is there large-scale unemployment in the sector despite concerns about overprovision [20]. Job numbers have fallen in some countries, but have increased in others while the numbers seeking to enter the medical and nursing professions have generally stayed stable or risen [21]. There has been some movement of employment from the public to private sector and there is increasing evidence of changing contract type. The statistics on numbers of jobs have not however, reassured the work force. All staff are aware of the pressures to reduce public expenditure and they fear losing their jobs in public service cut backs or because of privatization even where there is little evidence that redundancies are taking place (Afford, 2001). They are also conscious that if restructuring means an end to their jobs (whether skilled or unskilled), there are few if any employment alternatives available [22]. The introduction of markets in housing, utilities, foodstuffs, and other commodities all make health service staff ever more vulnerable to the erosions of their work, employment and income security. The shortcomings of the benefits system further compound the stresses health workers face since there are no adequate safeguards to protect them.

[20] The labour intensive approach of the pre-transition era invited numerous and persistent suggestions from international experts that staff levels should be cut significantly, regardless of the lack of capital investment to offset staff loses or alternative employment for those made redundant.

[21] Medical and nursing schools still operate selective entry procedures and demand for places outstrips supply in many countries, which has led private (poorly regulated) schools to open in some.

[22] Health services tend to be organized so to that there is one clinic per neighbourhood and one hospital per district (or at best one general, one paediatric and one obstetric hospital per district) which reduces alternative (local) employment options for any staff made redundant while unemployment outside the health service is higher on average in most of CEE and CIS than it is within the health sector.

Transition has meant more to health services however than a funding crisis, worsening pay and conditions and rising fear of unemployment. The prospect of EU entry for "countries in rapid transition" (accession states) is creating pressure to harmonize with western approaches to care. Similarly expert advisers (and to a lesser extent evidence-based practice) are promoting organizational models that may have few roots in CEE or CIS, without having consulted adequately and before developing any proper type of accountability [23]. The fragmentation and casualization of employment is undermining the ability of health systems to tackle system wide (corporatist) agreements on best practice and the shifting nature of employment and government and trade union roles has eroded tripartite alliance building on health policy. Public perceptions of the health sector do not help either. A lack of investment and reliance on out-of-pocket payments (formal and informal) exacerbate dissatisfaction with services which in turn contributes to a feeling amongst health workers that they are under valued and therefore poorly protected (in terms of popular support) from privatization or public service cuts.

On top of all this, the health system has also had to face a fundamental re-examination of the place of health in the benefit package. Whereas before transition, it was accepted as a core element of the provision made for society there is now a real competition for funds and for a place as part of the social safety net. How to pay for unemployment, how to cover the costs of pensions and how to provide social assistance all compete with how to pay for health care. Donor agencies the IMF, and World Bank are not against a public health service per se but they are promoting reforms, which raise the spectre of privatized social policy. They go beyond encouraging cost reduction to address resource collection, pooling and allocation in ways that threaten some of the basic assumptions (solidarity, equity and access) [24] that had guided health care organization over the previous 50 years.

The implications of health sector responses for health sector staff

The "context for health" is therefore a problematic one. The operating environment has changed radically and health is now in competition with other social needs. The way health systems have been configured is not sustainable, particularly given the rising costs of pharmaceuticals and new technology, the investment needed to counter the results of years of neglect, relatively high

---

[23] The DSE *"Public Service Reforms and the impact on health sector personnel'"* (WHO, 2001a) highlights the need for governments and international agencies to build consultation procedures into the earliest stages of reform and to continue to consult throughout implementation.

[24] The World Health Report 2000 (WHO, 2001b) recasts some of the core values in terms of fairness, responsiveness, quality and efficiency but the fundamental issue remains the same, whether or not people can secure health care based on need rather than on the ability to pay.

staffing levels and the wider economic pressures that exist. There is clearly a perceived and a real need for reform. There is however, little understanding of how best to translate reform models into practice and less recognition still of the importance of including in policy-makers' thinking the impact of any change on health sector staff.

Those attempting to reform health care systems (or advising on their reform) may occasionally have been entirely market-oriented but most often they have worked from the assumption that health is a special and value rich commodity that cannot be treated like any other entitlement or benefit. There is obviously considerable justification for this. Health and ill health are powerful determinants of quality of life. Societies often regard equity and solidarity as part and parcel of appropriate health care services provision in a way they do not when other services and utilities are considered. Similarly, demand for health, the nature of supply and its interaction with demand as described in health economics are somewhat special. There is a clear public good associated with investment in public health, at the very least in terms of controlling communicable diseases. There is also a clear mismatch between the time when people can afford to pay for health care (in the middle of life when they are working) and when they actually need health care provision {at the beginning and end of life when they are not working} (Normand, 1998). Solidarity is therefore seen not just as an ethical issue but also as the only rational way of spreading the cost of health care across a lifetime, allowing for the risk element, and providing for the potentially catastrophic costs of some health interventions. There is also a growing weight of evidence that health does play a part as a precursor of development and that without efforts to ameliorate ill health those communities affected will be trapped in poverty and will not be able to benefit optimally from economic development opportunities (WHO, 2002a).

Nonetheless, the unique elements of health and its role in well-being are not necessarily more significant than those wider determinants of health like housing, diet and significantly employment. It is regrettable perhaps that the experts advising on how best to structure and restructure health care systems focus so exclusively on the importance of health care services and overlook the significance of health care systems as employers. The concentration on mechanisms that are consistent with a health economists reading of the world have often led to reform strategies, which overlook the needs of the workforce.

Payment mechanisms for staff are a case in point [25]. There is an immense literature on how to combine elements of pay for physicians. These are regarded as crucial because they are seen as levers to control physician behaviour, which will ensure their work is consistent with system objectives and within affordable limits (rather than being an engine for ever greater expenditure). This is an admirable consideration but overlooks entirely what it is that a doctor needs to

---

[25] Consideration of pay does not include discussion of informal payments.

live on or how much they may be paid relative to professionals in other sectors. Most strikingly of all the literature focus on physicians reveals the lack of thinking about other groups of staff even though they make up the bulk of health sector staff. Nurses' pay and conditions do occasionally receive some attention, (often in the context of encouraging them to "substitute" for physicians), but analysts routinely ignore the importance of the socio-economic security of technicians, administrators and other support staff to how health systems actually work. They may not determine overall expenditure on health but must make an enormous difference to the efficiency, effectiveness and quality of care and so ultimately to the population's health.

It is typical that the focus on mechanisms and structures that might enhance performance should crowd out proper consideration of the people working in health. Decentralization, perhaps the most widespread (and most frequently cited) reform provides another, compelling example of this. It was almost a truism of health policy advice in the 1990s that to be closer to the patient i.e. to decentralize was to be "better". Certainly the Ljubljana Charter signed by the Member States of the WHO European Region promotes the beliefs that health care systems should be of the highest quality; that quality implies responsiveness to patients; and that being able to adapt services to local needs is part and parcel of responsiveness [26]. It was held that efficiency, effectiveness, and quality could best be delivered locally so post-communist societies were encouraged to break up the monolithic structures of their centrally planned economies and allow local management, devolution of decision-making and a mixture of ownership and organizational forms. Advice to decentralize from external theorists chimed with a strong desire on the part of many national policy-makers to reject the overly dogmatic, command and control approach of the years before transition. Opting to devolve authority was almost as an act of faith and a means of asserting a new identity. Some Ministries were reluctant to lose their grip and resisted but only in exceptional cases were they able to halt the roll out of power to local government. Decentralization was extraordinarily widespread and was intertwined with a number of other reforms. It was carried out however, with surprisingly little thought for how it would work in practice. This is not to suggest that centralization is preferable to decentralization. It is rather that it had huge and unintended consequences for employment, which do not seem to have figured at all in the deliberations of planners.

Crucially, decentralization has fragmented employment. It has seen employment contracts pass from a single employer to the level of the institution (hospital, polyclinic or single handed practice), transforming the rights and employment, income and voice representation security of workers. It has raised general problems of inequity within countries and between urban and rural areas

---

[26] The World Health Report 2000 (WHO, 2001b) confirms the sense that responsiveness is a key dimension for measuring the performance of health systems, but is less prescriptive in suggesting how that should be achieved.

in particular. The Russian Federation for example has seen disparities in pay between regions widen into an enormous gulf (Stepantchikova *et al.*, 2001). It also undermines the concept of equal pay for equal work (in comparable circumstances). Poland has cases of workers in the same hospital, doing the same jobs but receiving different salaries because they are employed by different levels of government (Karski *et al.*, 1999). Decentralization also threatens union membership and the right of staff to access collective bargaining since small employment units are not easy environments for unions to operate in. Crucially, it has also seen a transfer of responsibilities to local government (neighbourhood, district, regional) for which those authorities were wholly unprepared. There are enormous, and now acknowledged, gaps in the training and capacity of staff to take on new responsibilities and most importantly a huge lack of financial reserves and resources at local level. This has meant institutions and local government have frequently failed as employers with indebtedness, payment in arrears and under investment all dogging decentralized efforts to sustain reasonable security for staff.

Another common reform strategy has been the shift to social health insurance. It is distinct from decentralization but is linked to it in that it implies the passing of government authority to an insurance fund, often with a set of regional structures, which further deconcentrate authority. Nonetheless, decentralization is not its core objective. It was intended to introduce mechanisms to control output and efficiency and it was also expected to enhance quality by linking payment and performance. There was also a desire to achieve three further objectives. The first was to ring fence or protect plummeting health care expenditure. The second was (to be seen) to empower consumers. The third was to create a mechanism whereby patients could make a clear connection between the care they consumed and what they paid for it. Payroll deductions were expected to bring home to people what they put into the health care system, which in turn was expected to make them value the services they received. The move to insurance was not as "universally" advocated as decentralization and many analysts warned that health care financing based on general taxation was actually the most cost-effective and appropriate way to meet societal objectives where these include the provision of universal health care, free at the point of use. However, there was support in countries for any reform that was seen to emphasize the shift away from the past, to establish ties with a Bismarckian heritage and to align the country with Germany. The World Bank tended to support any mechanism which would allow for private elements to be included and that paved the way for clear constraints on what would be provided. Insurance is such a mechanism and invites the creation of a minimum, universal package supplemented by private and voluntary schemes.

To date insurance has not had a marked impact on employment within the health sector but it is beginning to make inroads into the security of some staff groups. Insurance mechanisms are ideally suited to fee-for-service style reimbursements (rather than to the reimbursement of responsibility *per se*) and so they promote a model of independent, self-employed contractors and single-handed or small group practices. Doctors are encouraged into what may well be less secure employment status and their support staff then tend to get moved out of the mainstream public sector. They work for the practice or practitioner instead of the health service and become dependent on their individual employer. It has also undermined other professions *vis-à-vis* doctors in certain countries. In Bulgaria and the Czech Republic for example, insurance funds have chosen to negotiate fees directly with physicians' associations, prioritising the needs of one occupational group over all others and marginalizing employers and institutions. This reduces the ability of mainstream health service managers to negotiate terms that will allow them to meet the needs of all staff. What is more voice representation can only be diminished by the decision of funds not to consult unions.

Social health insurance approaches also have implications for whole new groups of staff who are to be involved in the mechanics of contracting, standard setting, monitoring of contracts, invoicing and payment as well as in maintaining individual records and accounts. These staff may previously have been involved in hospital management or in the health administration functions of local government and in many respects they should be viewed as part of the health sector, particularly since most funds are quasi-public. However, it is as yet unclear whether they will be considered as such and protected by those remaining mechanisms for representing health care workers or whether they will find themselves without a voice.

Primary care is another area of reform, which makes perfect sense in terms of effective health care delivery but has not fully addressed the implications for staff. Both WHO and the World Bank agree that primary care and in particular family medicine or general practice, is the most appropriate way of ensuring cost-effective treatment, continuity of care, and an appropriate gatekeeping function to prevent overuse of secondary and tertiary services. They recognize that doctors taking on new responsibilities require new skills and have therefore helped support the design and delivery of training. There has been less investment in retraining for nurses however, and a tendency to assume that *feldshers* (an Eastern European model of independent nurse-practitioner) would move within the new physician led structures. There is also evidence from Poland that general practitioners given the opportunity to become fund-holders and manage their own budgets tend to reduce staff levels, evade tax and insurance payments, recruit retired staff in order to avoid making pension contributions, and generally follow poor employment practices (ILO, 1998, p. 20). Health care reformers have not adequately considered the implications of this kind of behaviour for the new primary care model and for the employees of general or family practices.

A final tranche of reforms has been that of privatisation [27]. There was, and is, considerable ambivalence amongst health policy advisers on this issue. Privatization (in the wider economy) is part and parcel of the restructuring and the shock therapy insisted upon by the IMF and certainly antipathy to state monopolies is inherent to much of the support given by the World Bank. Yet the risks to universal health care provision of allowing a fundamental rupture of solidarity (in the form of opting out by the well and wealthy) is seen as an immense threat by many including WHO. There is a clear distinction made between privatization of funding and privatization of provision and once again policy advisers tend not to concern themselves with the implications for staff of this explicitly health market oriented debate. So far privatization of funding has been widely regarded as overly precarious and countries are encouraged to retain a public collection and pooling of resources to cover the costs of (at least) a comprehensive if basic package of care. Privatization of provision or of service delivery is however, much more widely accepted as is private ownership of facilities. The ways in which countries wish to contract with providers of care both public and private are seen as tools for achieving cost control, meeting quality criteria and so on. All of the countries of CEE and CIS have sanctioned private sector pharmacies and dental care, and many have extended privatization to primary care, outpatient care and diagnostic services. Hospitals because of the cost and complexity of running them are still largely in the public sector and still employ the bulk of staff. In some cases the acceptance of private practice was ideological, in others it recognized the fact that services were being paid for out-of-pocket anyway but without any form of regulation and in others it was an attempt to capture additional funds that were just not available to the health system through public channels. The position of staff scarcely ever featured in the discussions taking place.

Although most staff are still public employees the introduction of privatized employment is a significant milestone. Like decentralization it fragments employment, only more so, and it also creates enormous threats to security. Doctors who become self-employed may work exclusively as contractors to the public sector, and so can be regarded as "not truly privatized" but their pension arrangements, working conditions and so on will no longer be secured by the state. Most importantly the staff they employ directly will be dependent on their continued success for their own income security and will be far more vulnerable as regards employment and work security than in mainstream health services. The evidence emerging from Eastern Europe also suggests that private employers are more antagonistic to trade unions than those in the public sector, which bodes ill for voice representation security. There are

---

[27] Privatization can be analysed in a number of ways. According to Afford (2001), its dimensions are given as privatization of funding; private ownership of facilities; privatization of service delivery whether profit making or not-for-profit; privatization of employment and contracting out or the sale of functions. A fuller (if slightly different) analysis, which addresses privatization of pharmaceuticals and the public-private mix, is given by Hunter (1998).

also a few, worrying reports of the contracting-out of functions like cleaning, catering or computer services in the Czech Republic, Hungary, Poland and Slovenia (Hall, 1998). The experience of contracting-out in the United Kingdom was that the conditions for staff and the degree of trust between employer and employee were severely compromised by this form of privatization. Many health policy experts regard the introduction of for-profit services with scepticism and suggest that the "owners" of health facilities or medical practices can only generate a profit through savings that threaten patient services. This must also raise fears that the security of the weakest employees will be jeopardized by the cuts needed to fuel profit making.

Many of the key reforms (decentralization, the shift to insurance, the introduction of primary care and privatization) have taken place as the result of rather inward looking consultations between health system experts (national and international) and health authorities, chiefly Ministries of Health. Health policy-makers quite naturally, place great emphasis on the way in which health systems are to handle patients and on how different reforms will affect citizens' rights. There is little evidence though that they have ever fully engaged with the issues of workers despite the oft-repeated mantra that staff are the backbone of the health system (and its largest expense). A telling example of this focus on health rather than employment considerations is the way that negotiations with trade unions have tended to be supplanted by discussions with professional associations, or rather physicians' associations. Governments have increasingly co-opted them (or been co-opted by them) so that doctors now formally manage elements of standard setting and regulation in almost half the countries of the region. It is not inappropriate for professional bodies to play a part in accreditation or for doctors to champion their own perspectives (although there is the potential for conflicts of interest). It is inappropriate however, for governments to sideline unions and deal with representatives of only one professional group (the most powerful) as if they could reflect the interests of other health service occupations. Governments and their international advisers have yet to do enough to understand the socio-economic security needs of all health workers, including auxiliaries, cleaners and cooks, or to genuinely involve them in planning and implementing reforms that work.

LABOUR MARKET SECURITY [28]

3

Full employment was a key feature of the centrally planned economies of CEE and CIS until the transition of the early 1990s. All citizens were held to have a duty to work and the state provided them with employment opportunities. Since the shift to the market however, state guaranteed employment has ceased to exist. The ending of guaranteed jobs combined with widespread macroeconomic failure, has seen labour market security across the region collapse in sector after sector. The health sector has been affected along with the rest of society and has witnessed significant challenges to employment levels. This does not mean that all the CEE and CIS countries have seen cuts in jobs in health. (In fact trends as regards numbers of jobs are very mixed). However, it is clear that the old certainty that workers experienced no longer exists.

This section demonstrates how numbers of workers employed, levels of unemployment in the sector and the hours worked can actually mask labour market insecurity. The data often under represent the scale of the problems faced not least because severance packages and welfare provision available to staff leaving the health sector are so inadequate. Statistics must therefore be interpreted with care and in the context of wider issues, including the use of administrative leave, attitudes of staff and the stated aims of health system reforms, if the actual insecurity that exists is to be understood.

In addition, the section shows that the position of health sector staff in terms of the labour market insecurity is complicated by the peculiar nature of the market for health, the "state desertion" of the health sphere by national governments, and the role of international agencies. Indeed, the interventions of international agencies and the thrust of health sector reforms may actually exacerbate labour market insecurity.

---

[28] The IFP/SES defines Labour Market Security as adequate employment opportunities, through state-guaranteed full employment, or at least high levels of employment ensured by macro-economic policy.

Job numbers, unemployment and vacancies: mixed evidence of insecurity

Counting the number of people employed by the health services is not straightforward. The focus on staff has consistently been on doctors and to a lesser extent nurses while other occupations have been overlooked. This has often contributed to weaknesses in the data on the total volume of employment. Nor is it easy to compare the numbers employed now relative to those working in health at the start of the transition process. Factors complicating such comparisons include the introduction of new national boundaries and a degree of population movement resulting from independence and/or particular conflicts; fluctuations in definitions of the various occupations within health (http//www.who.dk); and the continued involvement of those at pension age in the labour market. Privatization, despite being relatively limited, has also made direct comparisons difficult particularly since much of privatization has involved the shift of staff from state to self-employment (ILO, 2001). The small scale of the private sector in health and its poorly defined nature make it difficult to map accurately the substitution of public with private sector employment and therefore, the total volume of employment within the sector.

Despite these difficulties in measuring the number of staff in the sector, it is clear that there has not been a wholesale, region wide collapse in jobs. The total number of doctors per 100'000 population has fallen in relatively few countries and has risen slightly on average across the CEE and although numbers of nurses have shown a more marked drop in countries like Bulgaria, Estonia and Latvia, the CEE average per 100'000 population is almost static. This suggests that there is relative labour market security, a picture that tends to be borne out by a superficial examination of unemployment figures for the sector.

Registered unemployment amongst health workers remains relatively low in the bulk of countries. Increasing rates have been experienced in Armenia, Bulgaria, Moldova, Poland and Ukraine, but again "official" numbers are low. This appears to support a picture of labour market security but registration does not fully reflect the true scale of the problem. A range of sources indicates that the recording of unemployment is highly problematic, often because of the wider economic context. Numbers are distorted by failure to register, the use of administrative leave, and the increasing stringency of entitlement all of which obscure evidence of insecurity.

The IFP/SES programme has described the extent of discouragement in some parts of the region. (Discouragement implies that individuals perceive no benefit either in retaining a nominal link with their employer or in registering as out of work and simply disappear from formal figures.) It found that in Latvia in late 1995 no more than a third of the unemployed were formally recorded, while in 1996 more than 75 per cent of the unemployed in the Russian Federation and some 90 per cent of the unemployed in Georgia were not registered (Standing, 1996, p. 237). In Azerbaijan the "official" unemployment rate at the end of 1996 was 0.8 per cent representing only a tiny minority of the unemployed, while the Ministry of Economy itself estimated the actual unemployment rate to be running at some 20 per cent [29]. This can only be attributed to the fact that in many countries the majority of the registered unemployed simply receive no benefits (see also employment security) [30]. It is clear then that official unemployment statistics do not capture numbers without work in the wider economy, which suggests formal health sector data may also mask insecurity.

There is still more "under-registration" because of the resistance of employers to making severance arrangements. This is discussed in more detail under administrative leave and employment security but in brief, employers often prefer to keep staff on their books rather than paying to make them redundant. Staff then have little choice but to remain (formally) employed although they are no longer paid a full wage, because they cannot register as unemployed unless their employer releases the appropriate records (the employee's work book). Registration can also seem futile because of state failure to pay unemployment benefit and the negligible value of any benefits paid. In some instances the existence of residual benefits in-kind associated with retaining formal status as an employee, like access to health or child care or housing, encourage workers to acquiesce with employers.

Evidence on job vacancies tends to support the picture of a sector without significant unemployment but implies that changes are taking place (table 3). It is unclear to what extent vacant jobs were a common feature of the health sector before transition but 1990 data for the Murmansk Region of the Russian Federation indicate that for many occupations the opportunities available in rural areas significantly outstripped the numbers of candidates. By 1999 the excess of vacancies over candidates had fallen significantly particularly for doctors, male nurses and medical nurses. If this picture and the underlying trend prove true for other regions and countries then it would suggest that surplus employment opportunities are increasingly rare and that unemployment will emerge as an issue.

[29] IFP/SES Socio-Economic Questionnaire on Azerbaijan (2001).

[30] In 1996 of the registered unemployed in Croatia only 20 per cent received benefits. In Bulgaria and Lithuania, the figures were 23 and 24 per cent respectively (Standing, 1996)

Corrosive reform: Failing health systems of Eastern Europe

Figure 2.   Physicians per 100'000 population, 1990–2000 [31]

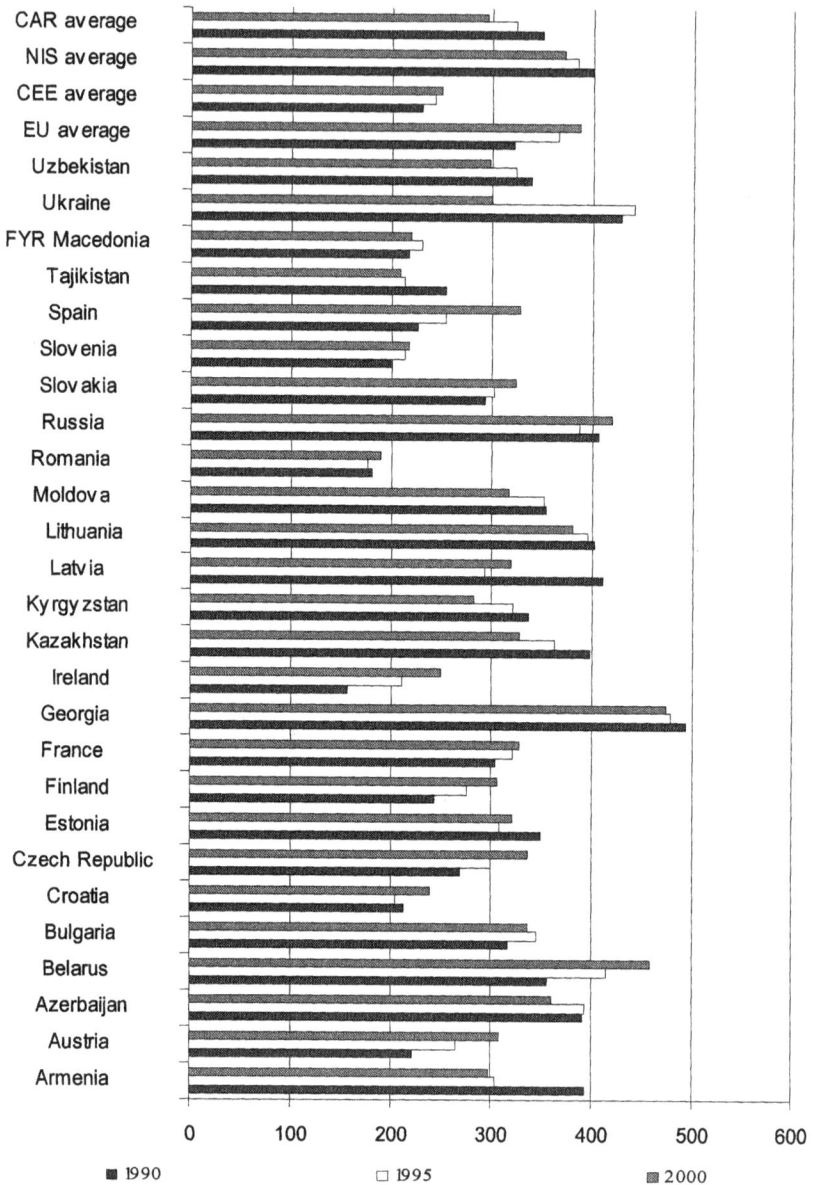

Source: (WHO, 2002b).

---

[31] The Health for All Database provides averages for central Asian republics within the WHO European Region, newly independent states and CEE. As before these groupings are not wholly congruent with those used in this Monograph but the data nonetheless serve to illustrate general trends in the region.

Figure 3. Nurses per 100,000 population, 1990–2000 [32]

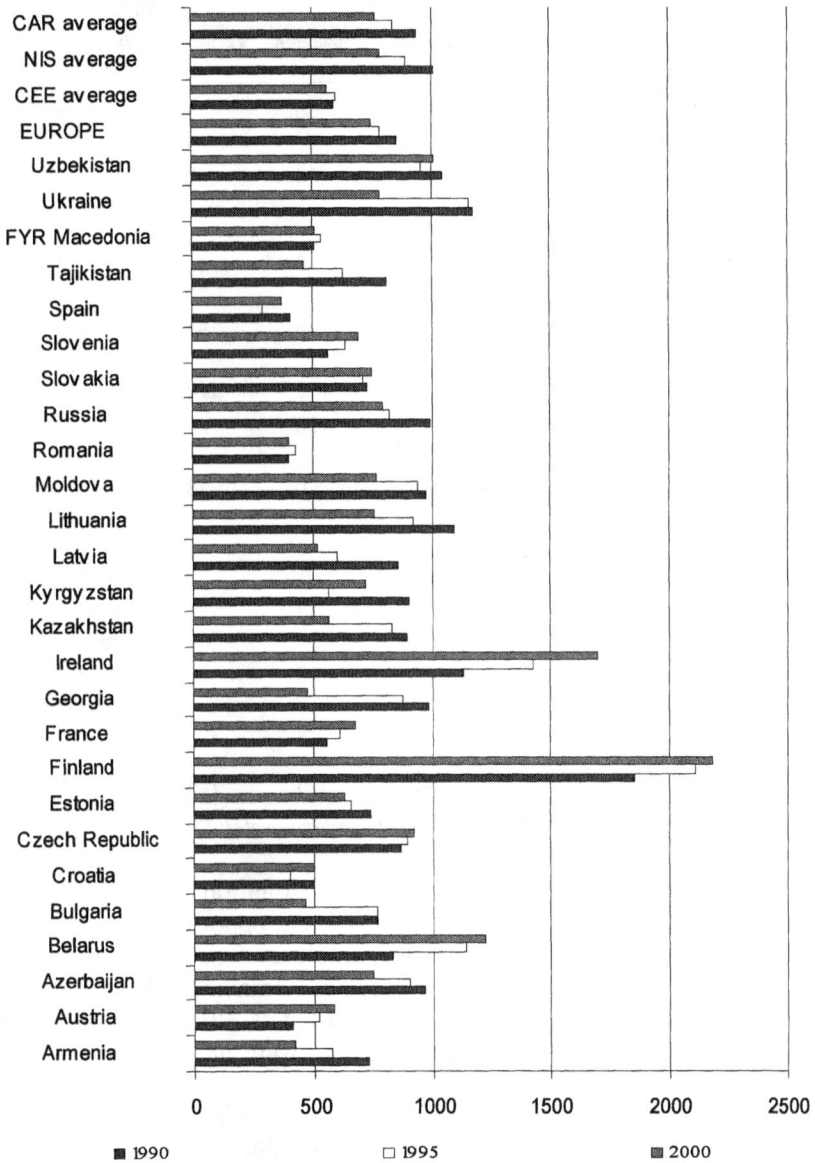

| | 1990 | 1995 | 2000 |

Source: (WHO HFA 2002.

[32] The Health for All Database provides averages for Central Asian republics within the WHO European Region, Newly Independent States and CEE. As before, these groupings are not wholly congruent with those used in this Monograph but the data nonetheless serve to illustrate general trends in the region.

Table 3.   Supply and demand for health personnel in the Murmansk region, 1990–1999

| Professional | 1990 | | 1999 | | 1990 | 1999 |
	Applicants	Vacancies	Applicants	Vacancies	Vacancies/ Applicants	Vacancies/ Applicants
Doctor	2	690	30	170	345	5.7
Veterinary	6	5	12	5	0.8	0.4
Obstetrician	2	8	3	11	4	3.7
Paramedic	18	96	36	43	5.3	1.2
Medical nurse	64	1'196	223	229	18.7	1
Medical registrar	0	5	23	5	No applicants (5 vacancies)	0.2
Medical laboratory assistant	0	6	0	18	No applicants (6 vacancies)	No applicants (18 vacancies)
Medical statistician	0	2	1	12	No applicants (2 vacancies)	12
Pharmaceutics	0	8	18	68	No applicants (8 vacancies)	3.8
Dental technician	0	0	5	0	No applicants (no vacancies)	5 applicants (no vacancies)
Male nurse	30	1'233	815	195	41	0.2
Total	122	3'249	1'166	756	26.7	0.65

Source: Informal data from the Murmansk Employment (Stepantchikova *et al.*, 2001).

The figures also hint at significant structural problems as regards the distribution of unemployment and employment opportunities. Again data for the Russian health sector give a clear example of issues that affect many other countries in the region including Moldova, Romania, and the Ukraine. In 1996 Russian medical unemployment was recorded as 3'000 in total, the majority of whom were nurses. At the same time there were many unfilled jobs with over 56'000 job vacancies for doctors and more than 84'000 for nurses (Stepantchikova *et al.*, 2001). These figures suggest plentiful opportunities and so labour market security but again the formal picture is misleading. Many vacancies were (and continue to be) in rural areas which qualified staff were often unwilling to move to. This continues to be an issue even as the pool of vacancies diminishes. Staff to population ratios between urban centres and predominantly rural regions are markedly different (fig. 4). Data for 2000 showed that only 8 per cent of doctors and 13 per cent of medical workers with a secondary education were based in rural areas in contrast with the 27 per cent of the Russian population living in a non-urban setting at the time. This has led to understaffing in some health care posts and the use of staff without specialist qualifications.

Medical staffs do not want to move to or stay in rural areas, not least because health sector conditions there are often significantly worse than in urban settings. This reflects a global problem and is particularly understandable in the former Soviet Union, where it is no longer acceptable to direct young specialists to rural areas and where no real incentives are offered to practice in isolated areas. Still, the unappealing nature of rural work compounds the unsatisfactory nature of labour market statistics, by effectively overstating the pool of jobs that are genuinely available to trained staff

Figure 4.   Uneven distribution of doctors and nurses per 100'000 population in sample Russian regions (urban and rural)

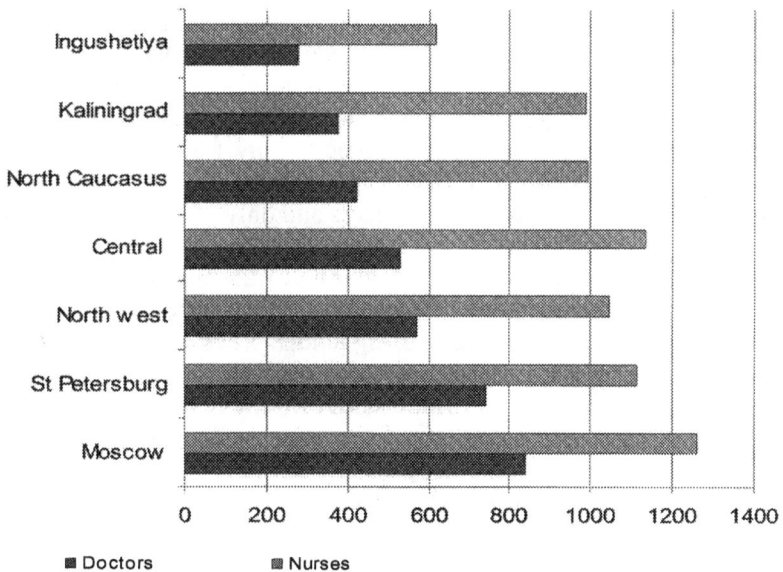

Source: (Stepantchikova *et al.*, 2001)

Insecure working lives:
long hours, multiple jobs and deferred retirement

Health sector staff work long hours however, in the majority of CEE and CIS countries their formal, contracted and actual hours have not changed very much since transition. With the exceptions of the Czech Republic and Russia where hours have increased and Lithuania where hours have shrunk, the length of the working day has remained a constant in the lives of health sector workers. This suggests a degree of labour market security but for the majority of workers the lack of change simply means they continue to put in consistently long weeks. Polish doctors routinely work over 60 and up to 90 hours, whilst in Latvia and Ukraine, actual hours for both doctors and nurses average 60 hours per week. Even in countries where the working day is kept to four to 6.5 hours for professional medical workers, (Russia), support staff clock up 68 hours in a week. The length of the working week is not however a key concern for workers or at least not for those surveyed in the Czech Republic Lithuania, Romania, or Ukraine who expressed general satisfaction with their hours (with numbers satisfied ranging from 64.6 per cent in the Czech Republic to 78.9 per cent in Lithuania).

Overtime is common in the health sector and increases the hours worked for most occupations (fig. 5). Its contribution to labour market security is complicated by the fact that overtime is often a structural part of doctors' employment[33], so 93 per cent of doctors in the Czech Republic and 70 per cent in Croatia regularly work overtime. Nurses appear to be in a somewhat similar position with 98 per cent in the Russian Federation and 65 per cent in Latvia working overtime. However, it is not confined to medical or paramedical professionals. In Kyrgyzstan, almost half of all administrative staff and a quarter of support staff work overtime compared to only 1.5 per cent of doctors and 5.5 per cent of nurses, while in Belarus 58 per cent of support staff work additional hours compared to 54 per cent of doctors and only 35 per cent of nurses[34].

It has been suggested, "the high rate of frequent overtime work in three of the countries surveyed must be taken as evidence of health care workers being over-stretched and/or facilities being understaffed" (ILO, 2001). In light of labour market and income security issues however, it seems more likely that it is a reflection of the need of health services workers to offset poor and inadequate wages by generating additional income. This interpretation rests on the assumption that overtime is paid or contributes to income generation, an assumption that is only partly borne out by survey data[35]. Even though employers may not always pay staff overtime, evidence on informal, under-the-table or gratitude payments suggests that working extra hours will increase the (informal) earning capacity of staff by virtue of extending their contact with

---

[33] Overtime for doctors is a routine European approach to providing affordable night cover and is justified on occasion, as a means of ensuring junior staff are able to accumulate sufficient experience to progress in their chosen area of specialization.

[34] ILO IFP/SES–PSI Survey (2001).

[35] In the four-country survey the highest rate of respondents reporting that they received overtime pay only rarely or never (90.8 per cent) was in Lithuania where overtime was the least common. In the Czech Republic, where overtime was most widespread, only 37.2 per cent of respondents reported rarely or never receiving overtime pay. Nonetheless, there was a marked discrepancy between the numbers often, always or sometimes working overtime and those often, always or sometimes being paid for overtime work.

service users. Certainly, staff surveyed did not regard overtime work as a major concern, which suggests that it led to adequate remuneration, through whatever route.

Although CEE and CIS staff tend to work long hours, they do not, typically, engage in part-time employment, despite some exceptions (most notably Poland which exploits this kind of flexibility to the full). This is particularly striking given the high numbers of women in the sector {79 per cent of the health services work force compared to 47 per cent of total employment} (ILO, 2000a, p. 17) and given the close association between women's employment and part-time work in Western health care systems. The preponderance of full-time work is very much the result of the extensive provision of non-monetary benefits in centrally planned economies and specifically the availability of crèche facilities throughout the 1970s and 80s. As benefits are reduced, the demand for part-time employment can be expected to rise, challenging labour market security. At the moment however, the ability to reduce working hours (and by extension income) remains out of the reach of most workers.

It is in fact more common for workers to hold second jobs than to work part-time in most CEE and CIS countries. The concept of labour market security does not easily accommodate the idea that having to work in more than one job is an opportunity to be exploited, but low wages often lead health workforces in CEE and CIS to that difficult conclusion. Up to 50 per cent of staff in the Russian Federation and 40 per cent in Georgia combine their formal roles with additional work. As is so often the case in terms of data on CEE and CIS labour markets there are no clear patterns or definitive evidence. Different occupational groups in different countries are more or less involved and the types of second job concerned also vary. Nonetheless, the phenomenon is widespread and cannot be ascribed to anything other than a need for increased income. Furthermore, second jobs are unlikely to attract pension contributions or to be taken into account in calculating benefit levels, and so, as with informal payments, they boost income only in the most immediate present.

Another marker of labour market insecurity is the number of pensioners who continue to work into retirement. This is not a straightforward measure of disadvantage as in the centrally planned economies, pensions were traditionally "low, paid at an early age, and paid on the expectation that most recipients would continue to be in paid labour well beyond the formal age of retirement" (Standing, 1997, p. 1350). Indeed, the percentage of staff also drawing a pension has tended to fall across the region (see work security). Nonetheless, it is clear that "market" conditions and the associated inflation have further devalued pensions in many countries so that they are below the minimum wage and impossible to live on. In Russia in particular, reforms of occupational pensions in 1991 left large numbers without the means to retire and forced them to continue in work. Typically too, those benefits that were paid were paid in arrears, sometimes months late. This treatment of pensioners will tend to undermine the security of staff approaching retirement or considering their long-term prospects.

Figure 5. Percentage of staff (all occupations) reporting overtime work, selected countries

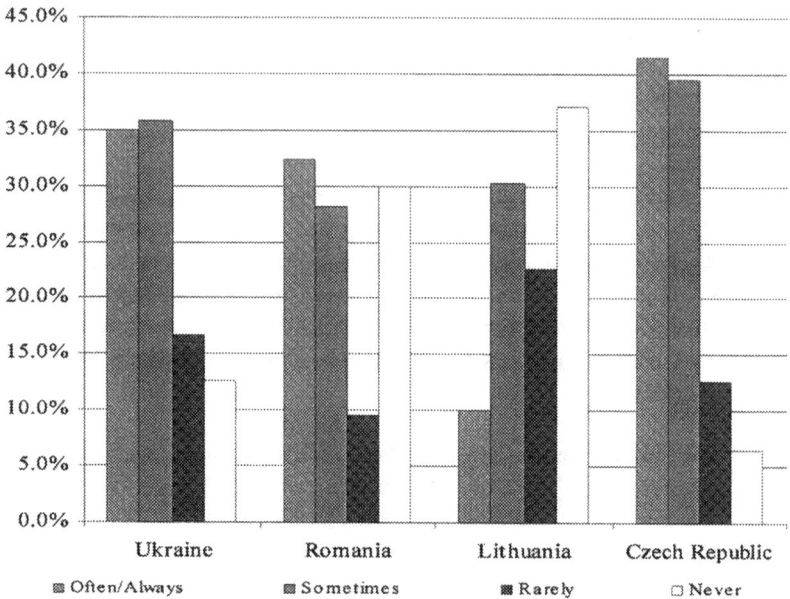

Source   (ILO, 2001).

Jobs that are not:
short term work, administrative leave
and emigration

Those CEE and CIS staff obliged to work after retirement or for long hours, often in more than one job may not be experiencing a secure labour market but at least, they are able to work. Administrative leave (whereby staff remain in formal employment but without formal pay) and short-term work deny individuals even this. Both are still widespread in the former Soviet republics of the Caucasus, Central Asia, Moldova and Ukraine. In 1999 for example, 20 per cent of health sector staff in Armenia were working short-time with corresponding cuts in pay while 50 per cent of Georgian health workers were either unpaid or only partially paid.

Staff placed on administrative leave and denied severance pay (as discussed above) do not simple quit their "non-jobs" and register as unemployed because employers often deny them the appropriate employment records (work books) to demonstrate that they are redundant rather than voluntarily out of work and because benefit systems are often hostile and inaccessible Standing, 1997, p. 1357). Indeed for many of those on administrative leave it is not possible to claim state support because opting to leave their "non-employment" would make them ineligible for benefits. Some staff do receive fringe and in-kind benefits associated with formal employment and, at least while nominally employed, they can retain some hope of taking up income generating opportunities (see also above on low registration of unemployment) [36]. Trade unions have voiced deep concern about workers trapped on administrative leave, their lack of cash income and the dwindling value of the non-monetary benefits on which those must survive. The conclusion that employment opportunities in much of CIS simply do not fulfil the needs of workers and cannot be described as adequate in terms of labour market security is inescapable.

Under such conditions it is not surprising that some health care professionals choose to leave the sector and indeed, their home country. Estimates vary as to how many people are emigrating, but the ILO/PSI survey suggests that some 25 per cent of redundant trained health sector employees in Bulgaria have gone abroad seeking employment while the World Bank has expressed serious concerns about the extent of emigration from Moldova (World Bank, 2001). Barriers to professional mobility still apply, although EU accession will lower these in many countries in the decade following 2004. Nevertheless there is already evidence of nursing staff being recruited by EU member states. Even where Western employers do not accept the value of Eastern European qualifications, it seems that pay for "lesser" or auxiliary jobs can still attract CEE staff. There is also anecdotal evidence of medical staff exiting their professions and accepting jobs outside the health sector in their home countries or abroad. Staff may be taking such radical steps primarily to achieve greater income security but unless the issue is addressed and incentives to retain staff are created it will become an increasing problem and one, which will compromise labour market security.

What fuels insecurity?

Many indicators of labour market insecurity appear, in purely numerical terms, to be relatively favourable. A survey of attitudes counters this impression. Trade union officials and workers share fears about unemployment and a profound sense of insecurity about the nature of the labour market. The ILO/PSI Survey of 15 CEE/CIS countries revealed commonly held beliefs that jobs were being cut and levels of unemployment rising despite data to the contrary. Privatization was cited repeatedly as a cause of job losses even where it scarcely existed and where there was no fall in health sector employment.

---

[36] Countries where in-kind benefits and enterprise based welfare provision have been maintained, albeit in a somewhat devalued form, are those, which also show a greater reliance on administrative leave (Georgia, Kyrgyzstan, Russian Federation, Ukraine).

Corrosive reform: Failing health systems of Eastern Europe

Workers' fear of unemployment must be an important consideration in understanding labour market security [37]. It is a new phenomenon for CEE and CIS, dating from the early 1990s only and taps directly into the reality of workers' experience. Some 40 per cent of workers in Lithuania believe they may lose their jobs within a year and 60 per cent feared they would be made redundant within five years. Almost as worrying in Lithuania, Romania and Ukraine huge numbers of respondents believed there was little possibility of them finding another job (65.2, 58.2 and 44.3 per cent respectively), powerful evidence of insecurity and an early warning that unemployment will quickly lead to a discouraged labour force (fig. 6). These fears undercut sharply any sense conveyed by the macro view of labour supply in the health sector that unemployment is not in itself a particularly significant issue. They are wholly comprehensible when employment opportunities in the wider economy are examined. Clearly, anxiety on the part of the workforce cannot be used as a simple proxy for labour market insecurity but the fear of unemployment coupled with the real lack of alternatives (paltry benefits for the unemployed, falling vacancies in health and lack of "outside" opportunities) strongly suggest an issue that is not being captured.

Figure 6.   Percentage of staff believing they have little possibility of finding another job

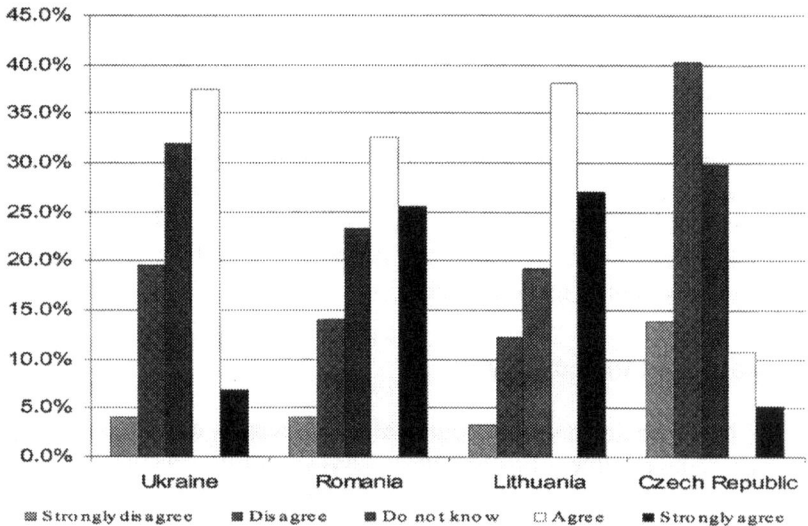

Source: (ILO, 2001).

The insecurity that exists is tangible (if not clearly quantifiable) and could be explained exclusively in terms of falling numbers of job vacancies, the extent of administrative leave and the inadequacies of the welfare systems in CEE and CIS, which make unemployment a truly frightening prospect. However, the

---

[37] Workers' fear of unemployment is examined more fully under employment security.

sense that there are insufficient job opportunities also stems (in no small part) from the pressures that international agencies like the World Bank (and on occasion even WHO) are exerting on health system managers to reduce job numbers.

It is ironic that while WHO emphasizes the role of the health sector in protecting population health and argues that staff are the most important of the health system's inputs, with performance depending ultimately on their knowledge, skills and motivation (WHO, 2001) it also advocates tightly controlled staff numbers. Similarly, the World Bank focus on restructuring health systems and reducing budget deficits has overtly undermined the security staff need if they are to stay motivated and deliver a quality service. The interventions and advice of both, and of other international and bilateral agencies, over the past decade consistently sought to reduce the provision of beds and staff which in turn undermined labour market security.

The pressure to reduce job numbers

It is a truism that ratios of medical staff to population in CEE and CIS were high, relative to Western Europe with an intense reliance on doctors. Certainly the former Soviet Republics had more physicians per 1'000 than was regarded as normal or desirable in EU member states. It is also true that the thought process behind the pressure for reductions in staff has an appealing logic. Reduce the number of physicians and you will not only save on wage bills but you will also cut the demand for treatment and drugs that they prompt. However, it is too easy to make selective comparisons between Eastern and Western Europe that ignore both outlying examples and national context (table 4).

These figures demonstrate a much more complex picture. Physician and nurse numbers across Europe vary more widely than the norms being advocated might suggest. Not all the countries of CEE/CIS have a high ratio of physicians or nurses to population while many Western European countries do. Italy is reported as having roughly twice as many doctors per 1'000 population (5.5) as Latvia (2.8) or Ukraine (2.9) while Croatia and Slovenia have a lower ratio (2.3) than Austria, Finland and France (3.0). Nurse numbers per 1'000 population are often more consistent with Western European norms than those in Finland, Ireland or Norway are (WHO, 2002b). Changes over the last ten years in CEE and CIS have also been more diverse than might be expected.

The "excessive" provision of human resources in the health sector in CEE/CIS is overplayed. It also seems that it is somewhat exaggerated. It is notoriously difficult to count staff in the health sector because distinctions between professionals groups vary, because the boundaries between social care and medi cal treatment are porous, and because of the way retired staff are registered. Data in the CEE and CIS often include more retirees than would be the case in Western Europe and the total for nurses incorporates staff that might more properly be regarded as carers or nursing auxiliaries. Those on administrative leave are also counted as employees although elsewhere they would be regarded as redundant. These approaches to data inflate employment totals.

Table 4.   Physicians per 1'000 population, selected countries, 1990 and 1998

	1990	2000
Belarus	3.6	4.6
CEE average	2.3	2.5
Croatia	2.1	2.4
Denmark	2.5	2.8(1998)
EU average	3.2	3.9
Georgia	4.9	4.7
Germany	3.0	3.6
Italy	4.6	5.5(1998)
Latvia	4.1	5.6(1998)
NIS average	4.0	3.7
Romania	1.8	1.9
The Russian Federation	4.1	4.2
Spain	2.3	3.3
Uzbekistan	3.4	3.0

Source: (WHO, 2002b).

More importantly still, statistics for physicians or nurses divert attention from total employment in the sector. Their numbers do highlight the significant proportion of medical workers to population in much of Eastern Europe. However if total numbers of workers in health and social work in transition countries are examined using the International Standard Classification of all Economic Activities (ISIC, 3-1990) then ILO estimates show that health services employment constitutes on average only 6 per cent of total employment in transition countries. This contrasts with a 10 per cent average for selected industrialized countries (WHO, 2002b, p.17). The difference cannot be explained by higher provision of social work services in Western Europe, although carers do appear in different guises in different occupations and in different establishments. The total numbers in health in Western countries are not adequately appreciated and the claim that Eastern European health services are over staffed must be seen in this context [38]. Similarly, pressures to reduce

---

[38] Health sector employment in CEE/CIS may not be disproportionate (given Western norms), but is nonetheless, of real importance. The Russian Federation has four million people in health (over 4 per cent of the national workforce), which gives some sense of the sheer scale of the sector.

staff, which helps create labour market insecurity, should be re-examined on more solid foundations. Certainly, there needs to be a better understanding of the scale of employment relative to Western Europe, of the importance of balancing different labour market indicators and of the implications of reducing labour market security before countries slavishly pursue further employment cuts in the health sector (ILO, 2000a).

The focus on physician numbers makes more sense if the experience of Western Europe (where supplier induced demand is a significant engine for health system expenditure) is extrapolated to CEE and CIS. However, this focus is less compelling when the actual situation in Eastern Europe is examined. Physician levels grew in the 1970s as part of a policy focus on epidemic preparedness. Then as now, medical staff were comparatively badly paid, not least because they were regarded as non-productive labour and were predominantly women. Low unit costs in turn fostered a reliance on labour rather than capital intensive responses to health care provision. These patterns persist because the continuing paucity of pay allows poorly financed systems like that in Belarus to hold onto medical staff and employ all medical graduates without straining the system. Given that pay is low and that capital intensive, high cost interventions and high-tech equipment are still not readily available cutting employment is simply not as relevant in CEE and CIS as in Western Europe. Again the determination to reduce staff should be re-examined with reference to the trade-offs that human resource planners must make in choosing between employment, activity, monetary and population based (normative) indicators (ILO, 2000a).

Different occupations: different challenges

The pressures to reduce jobs (appropriate or otherwise) revolve around doctors. It seems however, that they fuel a sense of labour market insecurity that affects all health sector staff. A closer examination of labour market issues by occupational group demonstrates that there are areas of insecurity for all workers, albeit rooted in different causes.

Doctors are not a homogenous group and while countries have attempted to control the production of physicians and reduce numbers over all some specialities have declined relative to others, reflecting population change. In the Czech Republic for example obstetrics has shrunk with the falling birth rate and as cardiology and geriatrics have expanded.

- Epidemiologists, environmental health experts, public health physicians and other staff of the Sanitary Epidemiological services have all experienced increasing insecurity as services have been reorganized and funding sources reformed. In many instances jobs have been cut as restructuring has taken place often in response to cost limits imposed by the IMF, although full data is not available (Shevkun, 2001).

- Dentists, pharmacists and some primary care physicians have experienced profound changes in the labour market over the past decade. Increasingly they are part of the private sector and are often self-employed contractors (or working in small group practices) with no formalized guarantees of future work from the state. The stand-alone nature of their activity and their independent status precludes any "cross-subsidy" between provider units that might otherwise support services (and professionals) in isolated or disadvantaged areas.

- Professions allied to medicine like physiotherapists and speech therapists have been affected by the economic constraints facing the region's health systems and, in some cases, by a shift to insurance systems, which prioritize only those services deemed part of a basic or essential package. Privatization of ambulatory services may also prompt a shift to self-employment or to sub-contractual relationships with fund holding or directly contracted physicians. Countries in rapid transition (accession states) attempting to meet the EU *acquis communitaire* are also limiting the number of recognized sub-specialties [39] and putting an end to areas like "therapeutic dancing" and "curative baths" with all that implies for the jobs of paramedical staff working in those areas. There is however, insufficient data to map clearly the changes in the labour market for these categories of staff.

- Paramedical and support staff jobs are also jeopardized by shifts of social care out of the health sector. This does not mean that jobs are being lost per se but that staff contracts will shift to new agencies. Data for the Russian Federation illustrate a huge shift in 2000 as the reform of social care took place (table 5). They also reveal that a long-term decline in paramedical staff per 10'000 population although it is unclear what precisely was taking place, or if this was typical of the region.

- Nurses numbers have fluctuated in individual countries (see fig. 3) and increasingly nurses are expected to comply to EU standards. This threatens the security of specialists in areas that are regarded as superfluous (as above) and poses major challenges for those who qualified in countries like Romania which had a "two tier" approach to qualifications or who graduated as nurses with very little post high school training. Finally, labour market security for nurses is challenged by the shift of primary care physicians and dentists to the private sector, taking practice nurse jobs with them. Nurses working in these settings are likely to be employed directly by the doctor supervising their work with their costs met from practice income. It is too early to measure the consequences of this change but it is probable that it will create pressures to minimize numbers employed and

---

[39] EU PHARE Romania report (1996). www.lshtm.ac.

bring down pay and conditions, undermining rather than increasing labour market security.

Table 5.   Medical personnel in the Russian Federation, 1992–1998

	1992	1993	1994	1995	1996	1997	1998	2000
Doctors total, in thousands	637.3	641.6	636.8	653.7	669.2	673.4	679.8	680.2
Per 10'000 population	43.0	43.4	43.3	44.5	45.7	46.1	46.7	42.0*
Paramedical staff total, in thousands	1'709.1	1'674.2	1'613.2	1'628.8	1'648.6	1'626.3	1'620.9	1'563.6
Per 10'000 population	115.3	113.1	109.7	111.0	112.7	111.4	111.4	96.5*

* In the Ministry of Health Care sphere.

Source: Ministry of Health Care, 2000, p. 100 (Stepantchikova, 2001).

- *Feldshers* are a sub-group of nurses peculiar to Eastern Europe who traditionally played a relatively autonomous nurse practitioner role. They were provided with additional training to perform preventative, diagnostic and therapeutic tasks, and played a crucial role in rural communities. Their labour market security is particularly under threat from imported models of reform, which would see them replaced by hospital-based carers (and this despite the fact that they represent a local model of the public health nurse advocated by WHO as a cost-effective approach to primary care).

- Staff of sanatoria and TB hospitals (whether doctors, nurses or others) are all likely to lose their jobs as long stay units are closed down in favour of community based approaches to care such as the Directly Observed Treatment Strategy (DOTS) for TB. It has been suggested that this will drastically affect the whole economy of particular "spa" or "sanatoria" towns but there is insufficient data to quantify the scale of the problem as a whole (McCarthy, 2000).

- Administrative staff might be expected to expand given a set of reforms that consistently emphasize the need for more efficient management and in particular information systems and in light of the fact that most countries are creating insurance systems. However, it is unclear how far current staff will be able to adapt to the demands of new management models or whether there will be sufficient funding to provide "non-front-line staff" with real labour market security. Nor is it clear how the decentralization and privatization of employment will affect the number of jobs in administration.

A lack of data makes it difficult to chart exactly the number and relative security of opportunities in the health sector for doctors, nurses, those in related professions or support staff, but all face threats prompted by the changes taking place.

There threats apply equally in the parallel health services that exist across much of the region. These parallel systems were the result of a political approach that saw health care delivery through the work place as structurally and ideologically important and sought to reward workers through services linked to employment rather than through cash payments (Standing, 1997, p.1344). Ministries of the Interior, Railways and Post (amongst others) and many of the larger enterprises funded and delivered a fairly comprehensive range of services particularly in terms of primary care and occupational health. Ministries of Health traditionally had little control over these systems and have had little success, post-transition, in incorporating them into mainstream change. Nonetheless, they are explicitly threatened by the thrust of health care reforms and to some extent by the shift to insurance. Much of enterprise-based provision was undermined by the economic crises following transition, some services were handed over to local authorities and others have been "deserted by the state" and closed. Although the evidence of how the staff are faring is patchy, it is clear that large numbers of jobs are at risk and that the workers in those jobs are not adequately considered by system planners. In addition, there may be significant long-term consequences for the work security of industrial staff if the specialist knowledge accumulated as a result of the close ties between the work place and occupational health services is lost.

The impact of decentralization, insurance approaches and privatization

There is little clarity about the consequences of the various health system reforms for levels of employment. Changes in management systems, privatization and restructuring are sometimes regarded as having increased job numbers and sometimes as having led to job losses (while the affect ascribed to the reforms does not necessarily correspond with the actual changes observed).

Decentralization has seen many local authorities assume formal responsibility for employment contracts and for paying staff without the requisite skills or resources to handle the tasks involved. Often they then failed to meet their obligations. It is still too early to say what the outcome will be *vis-à-vis* numbers of jobs in the system but it clear that many sub-national layers of government are poorly placed to protect or manage labour markets. Similarly, the social health insurance model that many international advisers promote has sometimes been at odds with workers' security because of a failure to attract funds or to manage them sufficiently well to underwrite job numbers in the health sector.

Decentralization and insurance have both encouraged individual institutions to issue or hold employment contracts in place of government and to review outputs and performance on an individual basis. Again it is too early to see how this affects the labour market as a whole but it does seem likely that it will introduce pressures to cut posts as well as challenging a number of other dimensions of socio-economic security.

Privatization has already been touched upon in terms of its impact on different occupational groups. Although it is not known precisely how many jobs are involved, the shift of pharmacists, dentists, primary care doctors and some diagnosticians into the private sector inevitably affects the security of the nursing and support staff in each private practice and is likely to affect job numbers. Privatization is not however, an all-encompassing phenomenon and the vast majority of hospitals and so the bulk of employment remains "public". Even staff who are now nominally working for themselves, or "privately", are often wholly contracted by state insurance funds and therefore comply with national norms. The exact balance between public and private should therefore be less important than whether workers operate in a secure labour market and whether the population are guaranteed access to health care based on need, and regardless of the type of market (state, private or non-profit/ non-state).

Privatization does however, prompt concerns simply because private capital demands profit and will naturally seek efficiency savings at a time when the health services of CEE and CIS and the people who work in them are already struggling. If greater efficiency means job cuts, it will be catastrophic for health workers already living at the margins and unprotected by barely functioning welfare systems. If privatization implies greater reliance on the contracting out of services and auxiliary functions it will surely weaken the security of the workforce, undermine trust and raise the spectre of job cuts as contractors seek to generate a profit (Hunter, 1998). This does not of course rule out privatization of services or decry the importance of private, not-for-profit providers. It does mean that the regulatory framework protecting the rights of the workforce will be particularly important if exploitation is to be prevented and staff protected.

Conclusions and policy recommendations

There is no clear, measurable, regional pattern of labour market security. Job numbers have fallen in some countries and increased in others and while unemployment seems not to be numerically significant, vacancies may be on the decline. Many staff work long hours and take on more than one job but others are placed on administrative leave or are paid in arrears. The whole area of labour market security is obscured by lack of data, uncertainty about what is happening in parallel health systems and the inadequacies of so many CEE/CIS welfare systems which make registering as unemployed all but pointless and help trap staff in unpaid, "nominal" jobs.

Labour market insecurity is not easily measured but is nonetheless a very real phenomenon as demonstrated by the fears of workers and their trade union representatives. International agencies promote cuts in physician numbers and in medical school places, and inadvertently generate a sense of uncertainty in all occupational groups. Many other health sector reforms are perceived as challenging labour market security although this is not their intention. Central governments for example, are increasingly withdrawing from health care provision, abandoning their role in favour of local authorities and insurance bodies. These "local" bodies may be better placed to respond to patients needs but they often do not have the well being of the labour market as an objective and do not inspire confidence in workers.

There are real issues about determining the optimum level of employment within the health sector, in the contexts of Eastern Europe. Shedding enormous numbers of jobs makes little sense if employment levels are not as high as is widely believed, if the cost of employing staff is relatively low and if the staff in place are shown not to generate significant additional costs. However, if low levels of investment are combined with efforts to maintain high staff to population ratios this will keep workers in jobs with poor pay, conditions and equipment and produce a permanent and vast working poor. The peculiar market for health reinforces these dilemmas not least because the greatest demands on the sector are often made by the poorest in society who can be forced into poverty by health system failures and because many in the health sector are already part of the "working poor" (WHO, 2002a).

The recent WHO commission on macroeconomics and health and its work with the World Bank have prompted an acknowledgment that employment contributes significantly to well-being and health. It is surely time to go beyond this and recognize that the interests of well-being and health cannot be best served by insisting on low state expenditures which can only result in low paid public sector workers. This is of particular relevance given how much of health service provision remains in the public sector in CEE and CIS and how important the motivation of health service staff is seen to be. There needs to be a re-evaluation of approaches to job numbers in the health sector and an active shift of focus away from employment cuts towards ensuring a labour market security that will maximize health system outputs and ensure that the health services play a positive part as employers. The following recommendations if acted on by the international/donor communities, national governments, employers and unions would help address these concerns.

International agencies and bilateral assistance programmes should explicitly (and actively):

- recognize the macro-economic importance of the labour market in health;

- acknowledge the influence of employment on the health and well-being of health sector workers;

- subscribe to the policy statement that job cuts should not be the initial, knee-jerk response to enhancing efficiency in CEE and CIS;

- promote research into the labour market in health with a view to analysing the cost benefits of different staffing levels and models of health care delivery;

- promote research into other areas of the labour market, and in particular, that of parallel health systems to establish employment patterns;

- initiate a dialogue with trade unions and associations on the structure of the labour force;

- sponsor and promote a code of practice for governments engaging in health sector reform (see below); and

- support the development of legal frameworks within the CEE and CIS that will facilitate protection of labour markets in line with the code of practice.

Governments should be asked to subscribe to a code of practice, which commits them to:

- introducing "employment impact assessment" on all proposed health system reforms (drawing on the approaches of environmental, health and human impact assessments), to map the likely consequences for jobs and staff of all structural changes before they are implemented;

- discussing all proposed changes with trade unions and associations;

- carrying out a financial and skill audit of all local authorities, health sector institutions and insurance agencies prior to devolving employment responsibilities to them with a view to establishing guarantees that the bodies concerned will be able to fulfil their obligations to pay and otherwise maintain staff;

- introducing legislation to protect job numbers and staff where jobs are transferred to the private sector (using the model of the transfer of undertakings/engagements protection afforded to EU staff);

- legislating against the use of administrative leave and the manipulation of severance entitlement by employers;

- addressing the welfare provision available and taking such steps as are feasible to enhance benefits, encourage the unemployed to register and prevent discouragement from the labour market;

- investigating the creation of incentives for rural employment;

- improving the quality of the recording and use of employment and unemployment data.

Trade unions should work with members and, where appropriate with employers and/or government to:

- collect and verify data on administrative leave;

- explore the causes and extent of unpaid overtime and its consequences for staff;

- seek to eliminate administrative leave and unpaid overtime;

- assess the impact on the labour market of pensioners' involvement in health services and lobby to ensure a dovetailing of benefits and employment policy that will protect staff whether they are entering or exiting the labour force;

- develop information campaigns to address members' fears about job cuts;

- identify and establish links with trade unions that represent staff working for other Ministries or enterprises in the 'parallel' health services and those that might best represent health care workers who are to move into social care provision or the administration of health insurance. Together agree joint mechanisms for reviewing the impact of reforms on the labour market, job numbers and employment rights;

- network across the region and with Western European counterparts to identify strategies to ensure labour market security in the face of privatization;

- engage in a series of debates, both internal and public, about the preferred balance between job numbers and health service costs in order to move towards a system that provides efficient, cost-effective and responsive care and decent, sustainable and rewarding employment.

EMPLOYMENT SECURITY [40]

4

The health sectors of the entire region were almost exclusively state operated until 1991. This meant that all staff were state employees and as such enjoyed a full range of traditional employment protection. This is not to say that health sector staff were a single entity but they were hired in line with clear criteria, could expect long-term employment, had rights that prevented them from being dismissed arbitrarily and were entitled to maternity pay and other benefits. There was a degree of uniformity stemming from the active use of norms in planning and management. What is more, as workers in the health sector they tended to enjoy a degree of employment protection simply by virtue of the nature of work in health services. The barriers to access to careers in health (for example the lengthy training needed to carry out medical, nursing or other technical tasks), the limited number of health care providers and the sheer difficulties governments face closing hospitals or health centres promoted long term, continuous employment with the same employer. All this meant that whether employees worked in highly specialist hospitals, the vertical structures of the Sanitary Epidemiological system or in small, rural health posts they shared a basic employment security. As the transition to the market has taken place this overarching protection has crumbled.

This section explores how real security has ebbed away even though a series of formal measures to protect staff continues to exist. It demonstrates that the erosion in the value of the benefits available to staff negates much of the formal protection they provide (although the provision of maternity leave continues to be an achievement) and gives further details of the misuse of severance pay. It also flags up the enormous threat posed by the introduction of new contract types and concludes that this must be an area for particular vigilance for policy-makers and trade unions alike.

Decentralization, changing organizational types and diminishing security

The health services of CEE and CIS include a huge diversity of occupational groups and staff working in different settings, including (now) staff

---

[40] The IFP-SES defines Employment Security as protection against arbitrary dismissal, regulations on hiring and firing, imposition of costs on employers, etc.

in the private sector. Nonetheless, over a decade into transition the majority of workers are still directly employed by national or local government and the bulk of them are employed in relatively large institutions (McKee and Healy, 2002). In the Russian Federation for example, even in 2000 most health sector staff still worked, for the Ministry of Health Care, and there were some 8'862 hospitals operating (Stepantchikova *et al*., 2001). It is true that there have been reforms aimed at closing "surplus" hospitals and beds but these are not wholly appropriate proxies for employment insecurity. A discussion of planned closures belongs more properly under labour market security since their intention was explicitly to tackle overcapacity and perceived overstaffing. More importantly, despite some significant hospital closures in Moldova and Poland most hospitals of any size across the region have escaped being shut down and some new hospitals have opened [41]. Similarly, where a reduction in bed numbers has been achieved it was often as a result of transferring medical beds to social care and so did not necessarily led to job cuts *per se*.

Despite this degree of continuity, there are a number of pressures for change, which have implications for staff. Decentralization and the reforms in the ownership and management of hospitals and health centres that this implies have significantly affected employment security, by introducing new forms of health care institution that challenge the traditional employment practices of the centrally planned economies. Only a dozen or so years ago health sector staff would be employed by the government and protected by the law regardless of how different their particular job or circumstances were. Now small, medium and quasi-independent institutions are springing up. Local authorities, autonomous institutions, private providers and insurance companies all employ staff and heads of new types of institutions demand "flexibility" in appointing and managing them from the examples below.

Private practices (including dentists, pharmacies, primary care or family medicine centres and diagnostic units) across the region have introduced self-employment and created what are in effect small establishments (normally with less than 10 staff). They are making decisions on hiring and issuing employment contracts in an unprecedented way and often with no clear legislative framework or regulation to support their efforts or underwrite the security of their predominantly female nursing or support staff.

Polyclinics and hospital outpatient clinics, particularly in the former Soviet Union, are experimenting with various forms of the fund holding model, drawing on the Kemorovo experiment of the 1980s. While the units themselves remain within the public sector, the clinic director is given rights to hire without reference to previous national standards for recruitment, to fire staff

---

[41] Evidence from the Health Care in Transition series suggest hospital closures were largely confined to those small in-patient facilities that had delivered seasonal social care to the older population, (particularly in central Asia and Russia). See also McKee and Healy (2002).

independently and to negotiate contracts with individual staff including agreeing incentive payments.

Limited liability and joint-stock companies are vehicles used in Armenia and Georgia to allow hospitals to remain in public or quasi-public ownership while giving hospital directors freedom from government constraints in terms of employment practice. Typically directors seek to use this freedom to establish their own local standards for hiring, firing and negotiating pay.

Convalescent homes, health resorts and spas are also being moved out of the traditional health sector. Some are simply being privatized while others are being transferred into an emerging public, social care sector. It is unclear how staff tenure is being handled in these cases or whether employment protection is being maintained.

There are insufficient data to give a clear picture of the extent of the changes taking place or their full implications for the staff affected. This is in part because the private sector does not routinely report the basis on which it works [42]. Nor is there any information on the training, the expectations or gender balance of the directors and heads of institutions who now control employment. It does seem probable however, given the predominance of women in the sector, that a disproportionate number of senior decision-makers are men. It is also unclear what is happening in the parallel health systems as other ministries and large enterprises carry out their own reviews of priorities. It is clear though, that creating a precedent that not all health system staff are treated equally is a significant step backwards for employees.

Certainly, shifts between institutional forms, changes of ownership and the transfer of employment contracts to smaller and less dependable establishments call into question continuity of employment and length of service and undermine acquired rights (ILO, 2001). Regular and secure employment is no longer a given (although there is no evidence on non-regular employment emerging). Who an individual works for is becoming progressively more important as employment rights increasingly depend upon the relationship and contract staff have with their local employer. Even where staff are not directly affected they experience a growing sense of insecurity.

This is the direct result of the withdrawal of national governments from the responsibility for provision and detailed oversight of care. Local governments have typically had to take on an increased role for in paying for and managing health care provision, even though they often lack relevant skills and are poorly

---

[42] In the Russian Federation for example private medical institutions are described as "not accountable to the structures of the Ministry of Health Care" and seem to provide (minimal) information about their staff only as part of the "periodic" licensing process (Stepantchikova *et al.*, 2001).

placed to meet their financial obligations let alone enforce employment rights. This transfer of authority has caused immense dislocation and confusion even where ownership of institutions and formal structures remain unchanged. Lithuania is a case in point. The Ministry of Health has stewardship of the system as a whole and shares responsibility for teaching hospitals, and for the country's public health network. There are ten counties, which implement health care policy yet it is the municipalities that actually provide primary health care. Employment is fragmented and it is no longer clear who underwrites employment security (ILO, 2001).

This begs the question as to how employment security can be guaranteed. There are enormous gaps in regulatory structures. National government seems unwilling and local government incapable of ensuring that legislation is enforced or that benefits, which exist on paper, are actually delivered, while there is no civil framework for pursuing workers' rights. Unless some overarching measures are put in place employment security will continue to fragment, within health system structures.

Duration of employment: a vestige of security

New structures and ownership arrangements may present growing challenges in terms of transferring contracts between employers but traditional health sector patterns of long-term service survive. Employees spend a significant proportion of their working lives in the public sector, within the health system and often with the same employer [43]. Data are relatively scarce and the use of administrative leave undoubtedly causes some staff to be recorded as long serving when they are effectively out of work, but nonetheless the majority of staff clearly have a strong and long-standing link with the health service (figs. 7 and 8).

This longevity of service suggests there is a degree of employment security within the health sector. It also reflects the prolonged training required to enter medicine and many of the allied professions, which tends to make careers in health a long-term proposition. There also seems to be an "ethical" dimension to working in health that many staff actively identify with and which encourages them to stay within the sector. It is also true that the transition years have not been easy ones in which to pursue alternative careers. High levels of unemployment in the wider economies of CEE and CIS may account for staff staying in poorly paid and stressful jobs, (although there is anecdotal evidence

---

[43] A vast majority of health sector employees in the four-country survey (some 80 per cent) noted that they had been in the public sector all their working lives. While this may be expected in former and recently communist states, it does suggest that there has been little movement between sectors since transition (ILO, 2001).

from former Soviet Republics that some workers are being forced to abandon the health system for better paid work like taxi driving).

Figure 7. Duration of employment (number of years) in health care reported by staff, selected countries

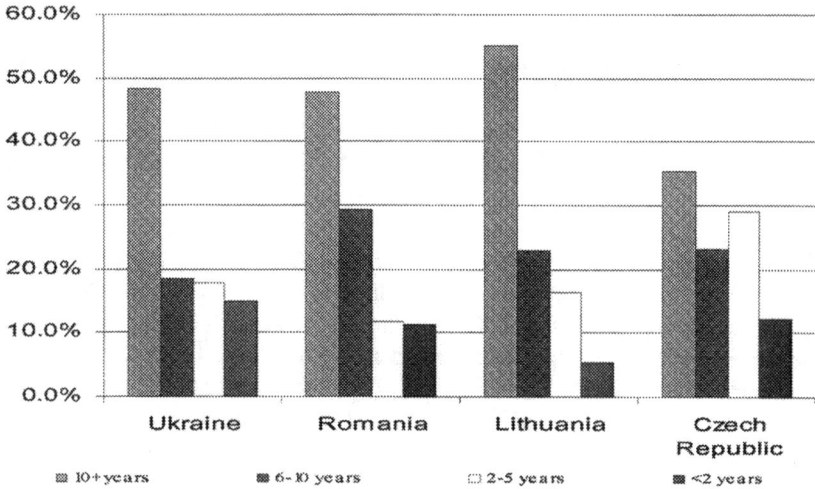

Source: (ILO, 2001).

Figure 8. Duration of employment (number of years) with current employers reported by staff, selected countries

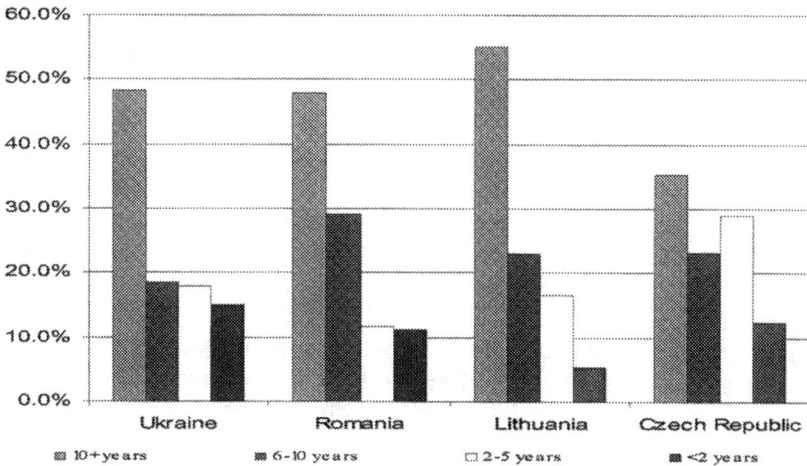

Source: (ILO, 2001).

The high average duration of employment in health is confirmed by survey work in a number of representative countries (above). The data also suggest that recruitment may have slowed in more recent years, except in the Czech

Republic, although there is no information on how the current picture would compare with the workforce age profile before 1991. The length of time that employees work in the same institution echoes this patter of long-term commitment (fig. 8). In Lithuania, Romania and Ukraine for example over 40 per cent of those questioned had been with their current employer for more than 10 years. The rate in the Czech Republic was significantly lower, but this may be because the formal employer or employing institution has changed as a result of a shift in ownership while the employee continues to carry out what is effectively the same job in the same physical setting. Duration of employment would therefore reflect changes in employment status consequent on health system reforms rather than greater mobility within the health sector *per se*.

The difference between total years in health compared with those spent with the current employer indicates some degree of movement within the sector. This may be lower than is typical in other areas or industries however, just because the scale of hospitals and the structure of health care provision create limited employment opportunities in any given area. There will tend to be only one maternity hospital or paediatric polyclinic in a district, for example, and this will constrain the choices open to staff, reducing their mobility and promoting long-term employment with the same institution. Overall then, the long average duration of continuous service in the health sector, and with the same employer, reflects the peculiar nature of health care, as much as, if not more than relative employment security.

The fact than many health sector staff have been in the same job for a decade or more does not protect them from the fear of being thrown out of work. These concerns have already been discussed briefly and just as staff anxieties undermine labour market security so too they call into question how far workers can be said to have genuine employment security.

The theme of fear emerges again and again across the region. The statement "I am afraid I could lose my job" elicited agreement from approximately 40 per cent of workers in Lithuania and Ukraine and some 30 per cent in Romania (fig. 9) while some 60 per cent of Lithuanian respondents feared losing their job within five years. Their anxiety is echoed when stress in the workplace is examined (see work security) and suggests strongly that despite formal protection from arbitrary dismissal workers do not feel secure. This insecurity is emphasized by the number of respondents who expected to lose their job (rather than feared losing it) within a year. Although rates were lower across the four countries, they still amounted to some 43.2 per cent in Lithuanian and 17.1 per cent in Ukraine (fig. 10) [44].

---

[44] Taking "strongly agree" and "agree" together.

Figure 9. Percentage of staff agreeing to the statement "I am afraid I could lose my job"

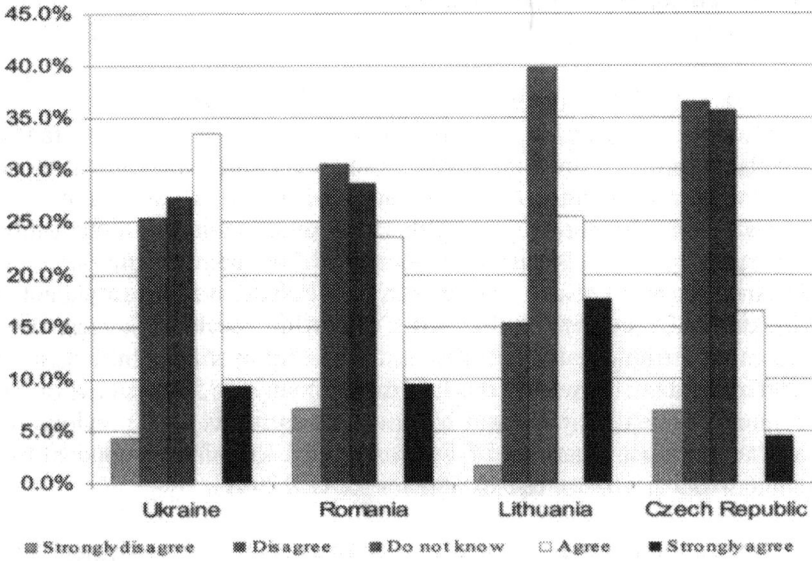

Source: (ILO, 2001).

Figure 10. Percentage of staff agreeing to the statement "I expect to lose my job within one year"

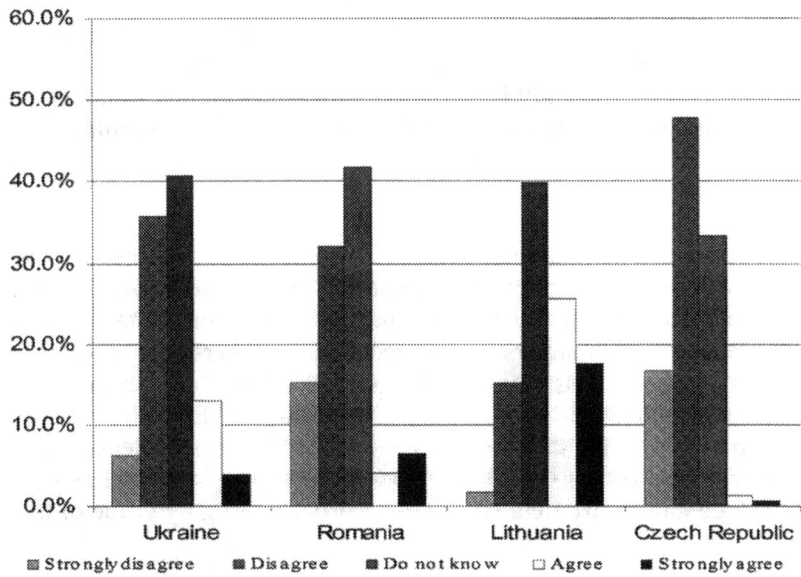

Source: (ILO, 2001).

Advance notice, severance pay and unemployment benefits: security in name only

The ILO/PSI survey confirms that the measures that ought to denote employment security, like advance notice of redundancy or severance pay for regular employees, are still in place. Both are a common feature across CEE and CIS, with most countries requiring advance notice in the region of two months and all those surveyed reporting that employees maintained their entitlement to severance pay. Levels varied across national boundaries, from one month's pay in Armenia and Latvia to six months' in Poland, and no respondents reported difficulties in securing entitlements. Again this seems to suggest that there is reasonable employment security and that employers bear the costs of making staff redundant. However, the fact that as many as 58.9 per cent of Lithuanian respondents felt their job had become less secure over the previous five years, and that almost a quarter of Romanian and Ukrainian respondents agreed, is enough to warrant some re-examination (ILO, 2001).

Severance pay is problematic as an indicator of employment security for two reasons. First, it is based on formal salary levels, which are frequently below real averages. They do not include any allowance for the fact that salaries are set in the knowledge that many staff receive (and in part depend on) supplementary under-the-table or gratitude payments. Nor do they reflect the loss of benefits in-kind provided through the work place, which have either been withdrawn without compensation (further reducing the value of remuneration) or will be lost on redundancy [45]. This means that the amount employers must pay in severance is significantly below what would be required to honour the spirit of the legislation in place namely, that adequate provision should be made for the member of staff losing their job to cover the costs of moving to new employment.

Second, and more importantly there is clearly misuse of the severance payment system by employers in a number of countries (not least in Georgia, the Russian Federation and Ukraine), which prevents workers taking up their rights. It is cheaper for employers to keep redundant workers formally employed than it is for them to dismiss them, so they keep workers "on the books" without pay rather than meet the costs of severance packages. Employees are discouraged from quitting by the threat that their employer will not release the employment or personnel records (work history book) they need to register as unemployed or to change jobs. Staff are also dissuaded from leaving by virtue of the fact that if

---

[45] In-kind benefits provided through the work place stem from the attempts of previous governments to replace monetary rewards with non-cash remuneration through services linked to occupation. They meant that cash wages were a poor measure of the actual cost of living Standing (1997, p. 1344).

they do resign they lose any prospect whatsoever of receiving severance pay. The possibility of securing severance pay may be remote but even the slight hope of a lump sum equivalent to something like three months salary is a very attractive proposition for workers who may not have been paid at all for weeks. This has trapped health sector workers in jobs where they don't work and don't earn any money {see also labour market security} (Standing, 1997, pp. 1357–1358).

Governments collude with this "withholding" of severance pay in many countries through their management of the benefits system. Entitlement to unemployment benefits is often strictly conditional, so that those who are deemed to have left their job voluntarily are excluded from receiving support, either temporarily or permanently. Workers on administrative leave who have not been paid for months cannot quit their jobs and register as unemployed therefore, as this would "disentitle" them to benefits. Instead they have little option but to stay with their employer. Governments allow this to continue because it reduces the call on public expenditure and keeps official unemployment statistics down (Standing, 1997, pp. 1360–1361).

Countries that have shifted to an insurance-based system experience additional problems because of the shortfall in contributions to the "employment/unemployment" funds. This lack of capacity to fund social transfers stems from falling levels of employment in the wider economy (and so of contributions); the privatization of jobs and the shift of work into the "informal" sector which has seen a widespread withdrawal of enterprises from formal insurance schemes; and from wholesale evasion. Governments have been unable to tackle this "opting out" or to manage contribution levels so that they generate adequate revenue to meet obligations without prompting further evasion. As a result benefits are not available to workers losing their jobs or to those seeking an alternative to administrative leave (Standing, 1997, p. 1349).

The failure of states to pay unemployment benefits inevitably contributes to the sense of employment insecurity. In 1996, 54 per cent of the registered unemployed with entitlement to benefit in Russia received nothing (Tchetvernia et al., 1997, p. 8). In Poland only 52 per cent of those entitled received any benefits and this figure fell to around 47 per cent in Latvia, 24, 23 and 20 per cent respectively in Lithuania, Bulgaria and Croatia and staggeringly only 13 per cent in Tajikistan and 10 per cent in Georgia (Standing, 1997, p. 1361). These figures are even more striking when the fact that huge numbers of the unemployed are not registered, is taken into account [46]. Nor are matters helped by the offer of some firms to pay their contributions as goods in kind, which on

---

[46] In Azerbaijan less than 5 per cent of the unemployed are registered, only 21 per cent of which receive benefits, thus less than 1 per cent of the unemployed are in receipt of benefits (Standing, 1997, p. 1361).

occasion have been passed on to the unemployed in lieu of benefits (Standing, 1997, p. 1361).

The difficulties in accessing entitlements (to severance and unemployment pay) and the erosion in the value of the benefits that are available have negated the formal protection they provide and have thoroughly undermined employment security.

Maternity benefits: intact but devalued

Historically, the region's planned economies tended to be pro-natalist and encouraged the reproduction of labour through maternity benefits and benefits in-kind, including crèches, free schooling and other childcare facilities. There were sensitivities about the different birth rates of the various ethnic groups within multiethnic states and on occasion particular communities experienced barriers to access to benefits, but on the whole provision was extensive and comprehensive. The entitlement to maternity leave continues to be an achievement across CEE and CIS. Women have a right to maternity pay in all the countries surveyed and all could return to their posts after leave. The duration of maternity benefits is often relatively generous and seems if anything to have improved over recent years, with only Kyrgyzstan reporting a reduction in entitlement to leave (table 6).

Table 6.   Examples of entitlement to maternity leave, selected countries

Armenia	140 days
Belarus	4 months of compensated maternity, with an additional allowance in the zone affected by the Chernobyl disaster (An increase over the last decade).
Bulgaria	24 months
Czech Republic	Usually 28 weeks at the birth of 1 baby; up to 37 weeks at the birth of 2 or more babies or if the mother lives alone; up to 22 weeks at the adoption of 1 baby; up to 31 weeks at the adoption of 2 or more children or if the mother lives alone; 31 weeks if the father taking care of the child lives alone or up to 22 weeks if the father takes care of the child instead of the mother; 14 weeks if the baby is born dead (unchanged over the last decade).
Kyrgyzstan	3 months (a decrease over the last decade).
Latvia	112 days or approximately four months (an increase over the last decade).
Moldova	4.2 months.
Poland	26-39 weeks (an increase over the last decade).
The Russian Federation	18 months (unchanged over the last decade).
Slovakia	7 months (unchanged over the last decade).

Source:(Afford, 2001).

None of the data from workers or trade unions identify problems in securing benefit entitlements and there is no suggestion that women are pressured to forego their rights. However, while the regulations underwriting women's security are intact and the leave on offer is generally good, there has been a real fall in the value of the benefits provided (Standing, 1997, p. 1352). This is in part because of the falling value of health care salaries (see income security), which reduces the worth of paid leave. It is also because of the reduction of provision of benefits in-kind. State and enterprise led childcare provision has often been withdrawn and where the loss of benefit in-kind was compensated at all it was often below the market cost of childcare and with benefits that were not indexed to inflation {Czech Republic, Hungary} (Standing, 1997, p. 1352). The various associated costs of child rearing in market economies have risen exponentially and the value of benefits offered to families has simply not kept pace with inflation. Furthermore, women on maternity leave are cut off from the informal (under-the-table or gratitude) payments that so often supplement their earnings, exacerbating the fall in income they experience. Nonetheless, what guarantees of maternity benefits there are, do contribute to employment security.

Challenges to contractual status

The whole issue of contract type had very little place in the health systems of CEE and CIS before transition and in many countries permanent (or at least long-term) contracts continue to be the norm for the overwhelming majority (fig. 11). However, there is some preliminary evidence of a creeping casualization of the health care workforce. The four-country study found that more than 10 per cent of staff in the Czech Republic and Ukraine were on fixed-term or temporary contracts while the ILO/PSI survey identified very significant rates of temporary employment in Bulgaria (20 per cent), Kyrgyzstan (24 per cent) and Poland (30 per cent) and suggested that as many as 80 to 100 per cent of Georgian staff were on temporary contracts. This would tend to put many of the benefits available to permanent employees out of reach of huge numbers of health care workers. The survey also provides disturbing evidence of the emerging use of contract labour and commercial contracts (as opposed to labour contracts). It seems that 86 per cent of workers in Georgia, 90 per cent of Latvian staff and 100 per cent of staff in Belarus and Lithuania are employed using these new contract types (Afford, 2001).

Some of this apparent shift from labour to commercial contracts may be an artefact based on confusion over terminology. It is credible, for example, that Georgia should have experienced a massive transformation in contract type because it has radically reformed the status of hospitals and the role of its hospital directors in hiring and firing. However it seems less likely that Belarus should have moved all staff into employment through commercial contract type as there has been almost no privatization and much else within the health system is relatively unchanged. Further clarification is needed of how terminology is understood and applied in different countries across the region.

Nevertheless, existing evidence does indicate a real threat. Changing the legal basis of employment and shifting contract type towards the temporary and the commercial will inevitably undermine the security of workers and reduce their entitlement to benefits. This will particularly affect workers in systems which devolve significant powers to hospital and clinic directors and those in small, independent provider units, where staff are already afforded less protection (see also voice representation security). Western European experience also suggests that changes of this type will tend to disproportionately disadvantage women.

Figure 11. Respondents by contract type

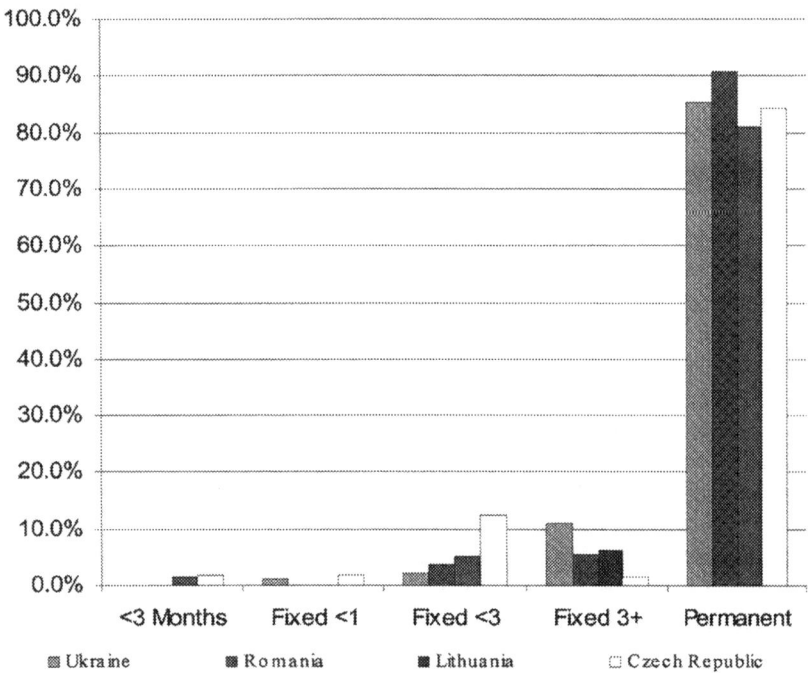

Source: (ILO, 2001).

Likewise, changes to workers' contracts brought about through the contracting out of services to commercial firms that operate outside the health sector will jeopardize livelihoods. Evidence from the United Kingdom on the impact of this approach suggests that the need of sub-contractors to make a profit exerts strong downward pressure on employees' pay and conditions and discourages trade union participation, which in turn diminishes workers' access to legal advice. It also tends to undermine the trust-based relationships and the commitment of staff that so many health sectors depend on (Hunter, 1998). The proliferation of this model of service delivery would constitute a major blow to employment security and undermine efforts to enhance quality of care.

Conclusions and policy recommendations

In some respects CEE and CIS countries have maintained employment security. The majority of staff have long-term links with the health service and are committed to a public service ethos. Their formal entitlement to maternity leave, advance notice of redundancy and severance pay is good, at least on paper. In reality however duration of employment is as much a marker of the lack of alternative employment choices as of security and many of the benefits to which staff are entitled are simply not accessible in practice. Indeed some are actively manipulated to prevent uptake, tacit barriers to severance pay being a case in point. As importantly the value of those benefits has plummeted undermining their whole meaning.

Security has diminished not simply as a result of economic pressures but in no small part because of health system restructuring. This has undermined the highly centralized organization of employment that was typical of command economies, and seen the growth of a decentralized and poorly regulated employment environment. Smaller establishments have been established, the directors of larger institutions have been given greater autonomy and local authorities have acquired more responsibility for staff (by default). None have a primary concern with the security of the workforce and most have few financial reserves with which to ensure that contractual commitments to staff are honoured. Increasingly staff must depend for the exercise of their employment rights on individual institutions and individual decision-makers and this has inevitably meant real threats to their security.

Health systems staff across CEE and CIS fear losing their jobs and clearly feel that the legislation in place will not actually protect them. They are pessimistic about the alternatives open to them and surely know that most welfare systems fail to provide unemployment benefits. Their employment security is therefore already severely compromised. It is further challenged by the spectre of changing contract type and of contracting-out. Both are poorly understood and difficult to map accurately but pose an enormous threat to workers. The shift to temporary employment, commercial contracts and contract labour (compounded by the poor regulation of privatized providers) will inevitably lead to the casualization of labour and will undermine entitlement to employment protection. The sub-contracting of hotel (cleaning, laundry and catering), information management or other functions will push staff out of the health sector itself and away from such protection as they now enjoy. It may particularly disadvantage women workers. Given the stated importance of staff in health and the emphasis reformers place on quality and responsiveness, it makes little sense to promote contract types that deny staff a secure future. It is surely more appropriate for planners and policy-makers to try to guarantee employment security in the changing health system context. The following recommendations may help address this issue.

International agencies and bilateral assistance programmes should:

- promote long term and secure employment contracts as the most appropriate for health sector staff;

- support a mapping exercise of the types of employment contract being used across the region;

- sponsor an overarching review of the legal underpinnings of employment protection on a country by country basis with particular reference to the implications of decentralization for security and to the actual costs of making staff redundant;

- ncourage the involvement of trade unions and professional associations in social dialogue on contract issues;

- develop a glossary of contract related terms used in CEE and CIS, and in Western Europe and translate it for use across the region;

- produce and disseminate case studies and analysis of Western European experiences of the contracting-out of health services functions; and

- recommend the indexation of benefits.

Governments should be asked to:

- survey the extent to which employment contracts have been passed to individual provider units;

- review (or participate in a review of) the legal status of decentralized institutions as employers;

- legislate to reinforce the obligations of employers to honour employment guarantees at least to the levels of those prevailing in 1990;

- address the status of those staff employed in small establishments ('single-handed' practices) by self-employed physicians and by the private sector and ensure the extension of employment protection to them;

- ensure legislation on contract type prevents the use of temporary contracts or commercial contracts as a means of undermining entitlement to benefit;

- commit as a matter of policy to allow the contracting-out of services only where a full costing of the options has been completed and where the protection of staff working as sub-contractors is guaranteed;

- map changes in contract type by gender, to ensure that women are not disproportionately affected by measures which diminish security;

- re-examine the levels of severance pay and maternity benefit with specific reference to the actual income of staff (where under-the-table gratuities are commonplace) and the value of in-kind benefits in 1990, and to index benefits accordingly; and

- take action to enforce the provision of benefit entitlement and to remove the loopholes which allow employers to withhold severance pay, trapping workers in poverty.

Trade unions should:

- track the numbers of staff being "fired" or made redundant from different health care institutions to identify whether particular organizational models (private practices, limited liability or joint-stock companies) or particular employers (local authorities, self-employed physicians) provide consistently less employment security;

- monitor the payment (and non-payment) of redundancy and severance pay;

- work with civil society to develop para-legal and civil structures through which workers can pursue their employment rights;

- advocate the payment of insurance contributions by members and employers and campaign against opting out of the systems that create entitlement to benefit;

- develop information packs, and provide support and legal services to those denied entitlement to unemployment and other benefits;

- present employers and employees with the evidence generated through experience in Western Europe on the importance of trust in the work place, highlighting the negative impact of new contract types on cooperative strategies within the workplace and on the security of the female workforce;

- carry out exit interviews with workers quitting the union to identify how many of them continue to work within the sector but are discouraged from union membership by the conditions attached to new contract types.

Job Security [47]   5

Attempts to reduce total job numbers and to move employment contracts to smaller, decentralized employers make the health sector environment increasingly precarious for workers across CEE and CIS. There are few guarantees left. Even the way different professions are defined, the content of particular jobs and the boundaries between them are being questioned. The technical skills and qualifications demanded in medical, paramedical and nursing work still afford staff some job security and protect career niches, but despite the specialization of different occupational groups they face a rethinking of demarcation and in some cases a root and branch reform of working practice. This has created a degree of job insecurity, unheard of before transition. It does not mean that all change is necessarily negative. The reform of the region's health care systems has created the potential for new skill areas and career niches and should offer a range of workers the opportunity to move out of the shadow of physicians and take on innovative and challenging roles.

This section examines the scope for development as health sector reorganization and reengineering of the workplace are implemented and as EU influence prompts a review of job boundaries. It looks at job expansion and recognizes that when the role of one group of staff grows this may be at the expense of the job security of other occupations. The links between job, voice representation and skill reproduction security are highlighted and the discussion concludes that job security can only be achieved in combination with other forms of protection, not least access to training.

Different rather than fewer jobs
— balancing the role of doctors and nurses

By and large the number of doctors and nurses has survived the "assault" of international advice. Public sector medical and nursing school places have fallen, but most governments have not implemented the significant staff reductions that the World Bank was insisting on through its restructuring

---

[47] The IFP-SES defines Job Security as a niche designated as an occupation of "career", plus tolerance of demarcation practices, barriers to skill dilution, craft boundaries, job qualifications, restrictive practices, craft unions, etc.

policies [48]. It is the type of jobs that health systems workers do that is under threat, rather than job numbers *per se,* and it is this reshaping of the role of different occupational groups that so compromises job security. While most CEE and CIS health sectors remain predominantly low cost, labour intensive and female, health system managers are increasingly focusing on the scope for adjusting the job content of the various medical and allied professions and revising the demarcation boundaries between them. Their interest reflects some of the concerns expressed by WHO about the respective functions of doctors and nurses and the increasing application of EU derived norms in an Eastern European context. It also reflects the expectation that, despite the lack of resources to bring about technology-derived efficiencies, gains can be made through reorganization within a labour intensive model. There are additional challenges to job security created by what capital investment there is and by the introduction of new approaches to treatment. The use of new technologies, pharmaceuticals and clinical pathways all beg the question, "whose job is it to take on these new responsibilities?"

The health policy-makers of CEE and CIS are working on the premise that there is a need to review career niches in health. Many have explicitly recognized that adjusting the balance between physicians and nurses could provide better quality of care and a more appropriate service mix without automatically increasing technology or escalating costs [49]. Certainly, the number of government-backed, World Bank or WHO sponsored initiatives on curriculum redesign; the uptake of EU PHARE grants on human resource development; and the range of bilateral agreements with Western European professional bodies in nursing, general practice and midwifery demonstrate region-wide interest in reworking professional roles.

The assumption underpinning much of this pressure for reform is that there will be some substitution of nurses for doctors in particular areas of service delivery. This need not imply wholesale cuts in physician numbers but it does suggest that doctors will leave discrete areas of responsibility to nurses while enhancing their other clinical and managerial functions. The opportunity for change is tied to the fact that before transition physicians across CEE and CIS were uniformly poorly paid and as a result were not treated as a valuable or scarce resource. They were often left to perform relatively undemanding tasks

---

[48] The pressure from international agencies to reduce total job numbers is discussed in Section 3, Labour Market Security.

[49] There is a correlation in West European health systems between numbers of doctors and overall system costs. More doctors seem to mean more tests, more prescriptions and higher expenditure. There is a danger that as CEE and CIS nurses take on more routine duties and free doctors for complex, clinical tasks, there might be a similar "inflationary" process across the region. However, the cost structures in a labour-intensive system if combined with controls on pharmaceuticals (through positive and negative lists) and on the purchase of high technology equipment would safeguard against this.

that might have been undertaken by less qualified staff in other areas of Europe. The part doctors played in routine, paramedical activities in turn contributed to the underdevelopment of the nursing role. Initial nursing education was premised on the concept of nurses as auxiliaries rather than as independent practitioners and little attempt was made to enlarge their responsibilities through post-qualification or in-service training (Saltman, 1997).

Revising this approach has serious implications for the job security of both groups. While doctors are unlikely to cede key medical functions they are being asked to hand over control of tasks that have been within their domain to "less qualified" colleagues. This will reduce job size in the first instance and invite the creation of "substitute" or additional tasks. These may involve new technologies and will certainly raise issues of skills mix and access to appropriate training. Alternatively doctors may face calls for redundancies. Nurses will also experience insecurity as they are asked to take on new areas of work and greater clinical responsibility. The changes anticipated, even where training is included in reform plans, may undermine the value of nurses' existing qualifications, detract from the career protection of current, overwhelmingly female staff and derail established career progression routes. Similarly, demarcation lines, accountability and indemnity in the case of clinical error are all called into question by changing job boundaries, further undermining job security.

The potential challenges to career or occupational niches are clear. The evidence on the extent of change to date is more equivocal. The number of nurses in a health care system is almost invariably higher than the number of doctors and this holds true across the region. Of the CEE and CIS countries with data available for 2000, only Georgia has a ratio of nurses to doctors of less than one and just six countries have fewer than two nurses per doctor (table 7). Most fall within the range of two to three nurses per doctor [50], which is broadly consistent with the balance in Western Europe [51], although total numbers of doctors and nurses are generally higher (fig. 12). While the relative size of the two staff groups does not say an enormous amount about how doctors and nurses divide tasks, it is striking that there were fewer nurses per doctor in 2000 than in 1990. This was despite efforts to reduce physician numbers and to shift job boundaries. It suggests that the position of doctors has not actually been unduly challenged by plans to enlarge the role of nurses since, in practice, doctors have

---

[50] Two of the six countries that are not in this range have ratios of nurses to doctors that are virtually two to one i.e. Estonia at 1.96 and the Russian Federation at 1.9. WHO HFA (2002).

[51] The huge differences between countries like Finland (7.09 nurses: doctor) and Spain (1.13:1) make generalizations about the West of Europe difficult. WHO HFA (2002).

become relatively more numerous than the very group who were meant to be taking over some of their responsibilities [52].

Table 7.   Number of nurses per doctor in selected countries1990 and 2000

Country	1990 Nurses/doctor	2000 Nurses/doctor	1990 to 2000 Change in number of nurses to doctors
Armenia	1.86	1.41	-0.45
Austria	1.84	1.89	+0.05
Azerbaijan	2.47	2.07	-0.41
Belarus	2.32	2.68	+0.35
Bulgaria	2.42	1.37	-1.05
Croatia	2.38	2.12	-0.26
Czech Republic	3.21	2.73	-0.48
Estonia	2.12	1.96	-0.15
Finland	7.46	7.09	-0.55
France	1.82	2.05	+0.22
Georgia	1.99	0.99	-1.00
Ireland	7.27	6.83	-0.44
Kazakhstan	2.25	1.72	0.52
Kyrgyzstan	2.67	2.56	-0.11
Latvia	2.09	1.62	-0.47
Lithuania	2.73	2.00	-0.73
Moldova	2.76	2.42	-0.34
Romania	2.25	2.13	-0.12
Russian Federation	2.45	1.90	-0.56
Slovakia	2.49	2.31	-0.18
Slovenia	2.82	3.19	+0.37
Spain	1.80	1.13	-067
Tajikistan	3.17	2.20	-0.97
FYR Macedonia	2.36	2.34	-0.02
Ukraine	2.74	2.6	-0.14
Uzbekistan	3.09	3.40	+0.13
EU average	2.65	1.94	-0.71
CEE average	2.59	2.26	-0.32
NIS average	2.53	2.12	-0.40
CAR average	2.69	2.61	-0.08

Source: (WHO, 2002b).

[52] The changes in numbers of doctors and nurses graduating (see skill reproduction security) will redress this imbalance over time.

Figure 12. Ratio of physicians to nurses, selected countries, 2000

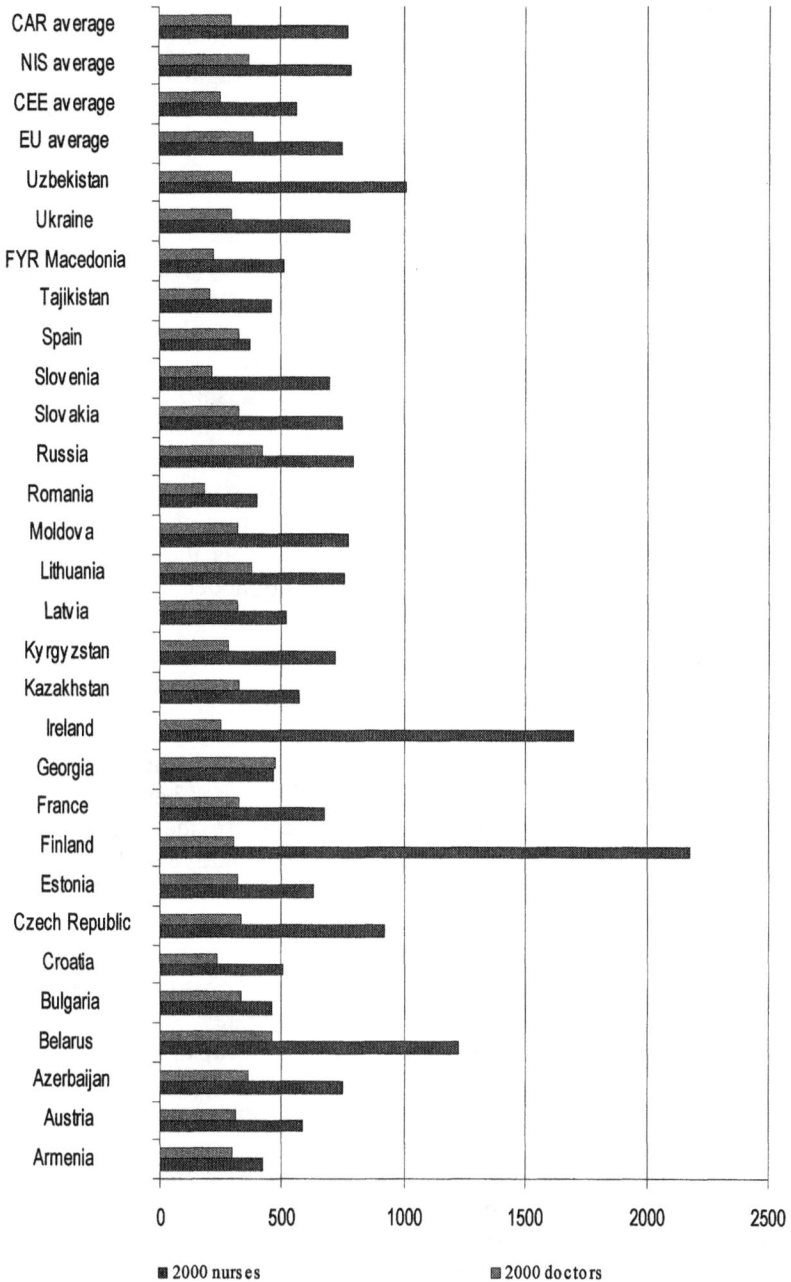

CAR average
NIS average
CEE average
EU average
Uzbekistan
Ukraine
FYR Macedonia
Tajikistan
Spain
Slovenia
Slovakia
Russia
Romania
Moldova
Lithuania
Latvia
Kyrgyzstan
Kazakhstan
Ireland
Georgia
France
Finland
Estonia
Czech Republic
Croatia
Bulgaria
Belarus
Azerbaijan
Austria
Armenia

0   500   1000   1500   2000   2500

■ 2000 nurses   ▩ 2000 doctors

Source: (WHO, 2002b).

Nonetheless, there is some evidence of change. Ten out of 15 countries included in the 2001 ILO/PSI Survey reported that nurses were taking on more tasks and particular reference was made to the development of nurses as a professional group in the Czech Republic, Hungary and Slovakia. It is no coincidence that these three are "countries in rapid transition". The desire to meet the *acquis communitaire* is exerting a major influence on the way countries are choosing to approach human resource issues in health and this includes the division of tasks between doctors and nurses.

CEE (and a lesser extent CIS) countries are ever more likely to use EU standards and norms as a yardstick in defining specialist areas and delimiting professional roles. This has led to changes in nursing curricula and training, which will surely translate in the future into new roles which supplant some of those presently undertaken by doctors. Similarly, it is likely that the diffusion of (appropriate) technologies and treatments will shift responsibilities from the domain of the physician to that of the nurse. Even though this change is slow in coming about, the security of doctors will eventually be compromised by encroachments into occupational areas formerly reserved to them. Nurses, meanwhile will have to tackle the insecurity that comes about as a result of being obliged to take on new skill areas and as the qualifications that were adequate a decade ago become increasingly outmoded.

Changing roles and responsibilities — the implications for all occupations

Health systems reforms are not, of course, simply about doctors and nurses. Nor can a general discussion of how work is divided between the two groups in a hospital or polyclinic setting begin to capture the threat change poses to individual occupations within medicine or nursing as a whole, let alone in other occupations.

Staff, taken as a single undifferentiated group, has seen an increase in the number of job tasks they have to carry out in almost the entire region, while in some countries the categories of jobs undertaken have also been upgraded (Afford, 2001). When the job content of all occupations was examined in the four-country survey, between 20 and 50 per cent of staff reported having experienced changes in their job tasks over the previous five years (fig. 13).

These data suggest that the job security of many staff may be relatively unaffected by recent reforms. There are some specialities and occupational niches however, which are particularly vulnerable to change. They often evolved nationally or regionally or in response to the circumstances of the Semashko system and are now threatened by new approaches to health care delivery and by a reallocation of job tasks (see also labour market security) [53].

Figure 13. Percentage of staff (all occupations) believing their job tasks were not changed over the previous five years

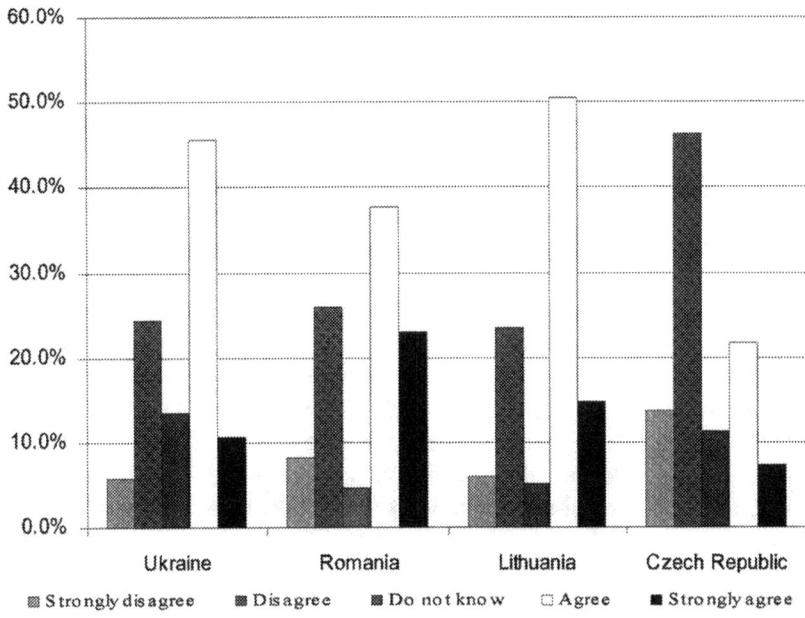

Source: (ILO, 2001).

The most obvious example is the *feldsher*, a type of nurse practitioner established in the Soviet era as a means of delivering a range of care to rural areas. *Feldshers* were almost without exception female, had one year's additional training and functioned as midwives, public health nurses and primary care providers. The pressure to comply with international standards and the increasing emphasis on technical, hospital-based skills threatens the very existence of this group, despite the difficulties often associated in recruiting staff to rural areas and the appropriateness of nurse-led care in these settings (Stepantchikova *et al.*, 2001). *Feldshers* are likely to face absorption into a changed service delivery structure which will demand the inclusion of different tasks within their jobs and the exclusion of other areas of responsibility whether this is appropriate or not. The introduction of EU style lists of recognized specialities and sub-specialities has brought about the "de-recognition" of traditional or locally developed medical practices, like hydrotherapy treatments or dance therapies based within health care systems. This bodes ill for the medical and paramedical staff who worked in spas, convalescent homes,

[53] The Semashko model with its heavy reliance on norms and it combination of residential and workplace based health care provision is described further in Section 2, Context.

"rehabilitative" units, long-stay TB sanatoria and other areas (the equivalent of crafts) that do not feature in mainstream Western medicine. They face the "deletion" of their particular career niches, and although some may see their jobs transferred to the social care sector many will undoubtedly face a complete reworking of what they do or the loss of their jobs.

Better-recognized occupational groups, including many of the professions allied to medicine and paramedical staff such as physiotherapists, medical technicians, radiographers, statisticians and laboratory staff have greater job security. Nonetheless, efforts to meet EU standards affect them too and often they must meet demands for new demarcation and working practices and for new qualifications. This inevitably creates insecurity, particularly where access to training is uncertain and when the introduction of new technologies is seen to favour younger staff or new entrants into the professions.

However, the environment is not exclusively composed of threats. Health services restructuring, the introduction of quasi-market mechanisms, the shift to insurance systems and even privatization have also created a demand for new skills and opened up new career niches in a variety of non-medical areas. While senior management positions still seem to be reserved for doctors, and often for male doctors (despite the predominance of women physicians), the need for accounting, financial and computing skills have paved the way for new types of administrative and managerial jobs. Again this presents opportunities for staff to follow new career routes, while at the same time threatening the job security of those whose existing niche is at odds with EU norms or who find new information technologies eroding their skill area, or who simply cannot make the transition from the old style of working to the new.

Coping with change
— rebuilding security

Many staff are expected to change the categories and mix of tasks they are involved in as the health sector environment itself changes. However, developing appropriate strategies to maintain job security in the face of this change is complicated by a lack of occupation specific, gender related or qualitative data. It is easier to identify broadly the opportunities for staff and threats to job security than it is to uncover details of who does what, or of how reforms that affect labour market or employment security impact on the division of tasks. It is clear, for example, that changes in job boundaries prompt fears of job losses and contribute to stress and insecurity but there are no data for tenure in any given job, and little evidence to suggest that changes in job content actually affect length of service. Average duration of tenure is still over five years in most cases and demonstrates that staff have long standing links not only with their current employer but with the health sector as a whole (see employment security). Nor does emerging evidence on the decentralization of employment and the increasing use of temporary and commercial contracts show any direct link to compromises in job security. Nonetheless, the creeping casualization of employment must inevitably undermine the ability of staff to define their occupational niche and where its boundaries lie or to specify what barriers will be put in place to protect it.

The evidence on the impact of organizational restructuring on the jobs of individuals (fig. 14) is also inconclusive. In Lithuania most workers questioned agreed that their job tasks were relatively unchanged yet they still reported in large numbers that their jobs had been affected by profound reorganization. At the same time Czech responses showed changes in their tasks were not dependent on organizational reform. This suggests both that it is possible to adapt job tasks and even job categories within a stable, relatively unchanging organizational setting and that the radical restructuring of institutions can still leave the content of people's jobs pretty much intact.

Figure 14. Percentage of staff (all occupations) believing their job had been affected by massive organizational restructuring

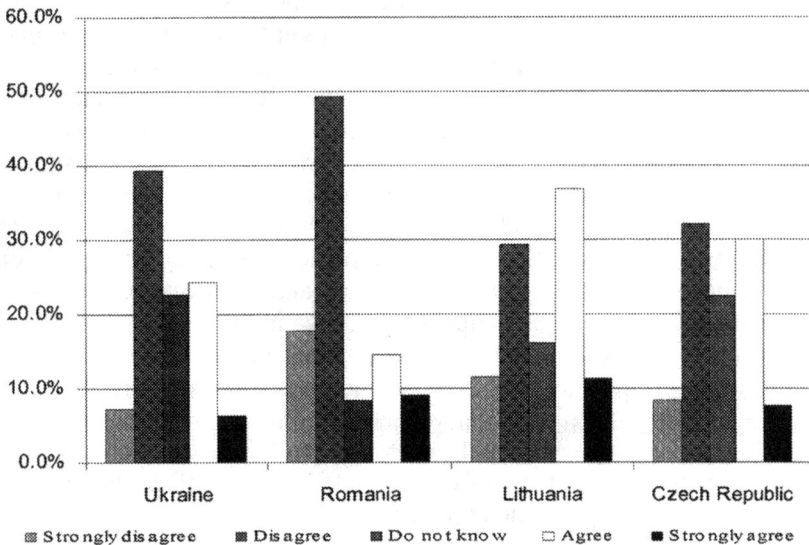

Source: (ILO, 2001).

Change is not therefore inherently inimical to security. Even though there are occupations that are likely to disappear as a result of a reworking of job boundaries, redefining roles does not automatically mean an end to long-term employment or a downgrading of contract type. Insecurity enters into the equation where there is inadequate consideration of the rights of workers and their training needs and when they are asked to take on new roles without adequate consultation, dialogue or sharing of information. Where workers and their representatives are not included in the development and implementation of proposed changes, reforms take on a negative dimension and will be at odds with security. Managing the process whereby staff move into a new generation of enlarged or altered jobs must be handled with consideration. This is particularly important because such a large proportion of the workers in the health sector are women. If adjusting job content or tasks were to imply shifting tenure or changing contract type this could jeopardize their entitlement to benefits, including maternity leave, and undercut their ability to develop a sustained and meaningful career. There are two essential strategies, which are key to ensuring that change does not mean an end to job security. The first is training and the second the insistence on a collective voice in negotiating the implementation of reforms.

Training and continuing education provide a route to security because so much of job insecurity in the health sectors of CEE and CIS is linked to job expansion. As jobs develop, staff experience pressures to acquire new skills, which may be understood as undermining their ability to fill their (new) career niches. However, if appropriate and effective training is made widely available, change can be appreciated as an opportunity and not a threat. This means providing existing (qualified) staff with sufficient skills to take on new job tasks and also entails adapting continuing education to ensure staff can maintain the skills they need to occupy new career niches. Traditionally continuing medical education was targeted at doctors and was mostly about "mandated attendance at periodic, post-qualification courses", which triggered incremental increases in pay (see skill reproduction security). Attendance was therefore assured, regardless of whether the training was useful to the employee or not (or indeed whether it fulfilled a health service need or not). This system has fallen into disuse. It needs to be replaced by a comprehensive and effective approach to in-service development linked to accreditation and certification systems which will allow members of all the occupational groups in the health sector to protect and maintain their professional or occupational status, and which will ensure competence to practice. Trade unions and professional associations clearly have a role to play in agreeing approaches to human resource development that protect job security. The balance to be struck is one that ensures that good reforms do not fall for want of trained staff and that staff in their turn do not fail for the want of adequate and appropriate retraining.

While for many occupations there is enormous scope for growth in terms of job content there are also legitimate grounds for concern as job boundaries are revised. A collective voice through trade unions or associations will be important in addressing those threats to job security that relate to job erosion rather than job expansion. In the case of doctors, there may be some fear that their position is threatened by less qualified staff crossing demarcation lines to take on greater clinical responsibilities. There is also likely to be a perceived threat from new entrants to the professions trained in light of EU norms and standards, leapfrogging over staff with more outdated skills. This will tend to be most challenging for those generations of nurses who were accepted into nursing school at 16+ and graduated after only two years, who are already less qualified than many of their colleagues. New graduates pose a particular threat to staff in countries that have not yet established a *numerus clausus* system to restrict numbers entering the medical and nursing professions, where well-qualified new entrants chasing limited jobs can flood the market. The problem is exacerbated in countries with unregulated, private nursing and medical schools that are willing to take on and graduate students without reference to the impact on the bargaining power of existing staff (Afford, 2001). Again a collective voice will be key in lobbying for appropriate measures to restrict access to medical and allied professions, particularly through unregulated routes.

Trade unions and associations have a vital role therefore as guarantors of security. They ought to be routinely involved by government and employers in addressing changes in job content; designing the steps needed to help staff adapt to reform; and thinking through the long-term implications of a shift to more flexible career patterns for both men and women. Furthermore they should insist that their voice is heard when it comes to tackling the regulation of numbers entering medical and paramedical professions and in determining the balance between supply and demand for staff since this will ultimately affect wages, bargaining power and career protection. They also have a crucial part to play in ensuring equal access to training and in-service development across the board and in securing the recognition and portability of qualifications. More centrally still, unions and associations are key to the establishment and protection of the norms that underwrite job security for all the various occupational groups within the health sector.

Evidence to date, suggests however that there are grounds for concern, as increasing numbers of CEE and CIS governments establish closer ties with professional associations, often at the expense of trade unions. The brief of an association is very particular, to address the concerns of one occupational group, most commonly doctors. Their appeal is considerable (see voice representation security) and has been bolstered by the willingness of some employers and insurance funds to negotiate directly with physicians' chambers. The sectional interests of physicians are given additional weight by the ever more commonplace decision on the part of Ministries of Health to involve their associations in professional standard setting, certification and accreditation (Stepantchikova *et al.*, 2001) [54].

The role of associations need not however, be at odds with that of trade unions. The benefits of allowing an institutional role for experts to help shape decision-making on technical matters are to be welcomed and should ensure reforms are compatible with the needs of patients and professionals. However, there must be concerns that doctors are securing a voice for themselves at the

---

[54] Countries involving doctors and medical societies in standard setting and licensing include Bulgaria, Croatia, Georgia, Latvia, Poland, the Russian Federation and Slovakia (Afford, 2001).

expense of other occupational groups and that the gender profile of the leadership of associations is at odds with the gender balance of the medical professions as a whole. Nursing and midwifery associations are emerging, but there is little evidence of their being given a significant, formal role. If governments privilege societies and associations that exclusively represent doctors then the focus of development in health systems will inevitably be skewed away from the majority of workers in the sector. Lobbying on demarcation, skill dilution and professional boundaries will reflect only a narrow set of concerns and the job security of millions may be harmed, detracting from patient care, and ultimately damaging the overall process of reform. The need to maintain and enhance links with trade unions is clear.

Conclusions and policy recommendations

Health service staff maintain a relatively high degree of job security because many occupations are distinct by virtue of their technical content (see employment security). A hospital pharmacist or a physiotherapist cannot simply switch jobs and neither one can be replaced by a new recruit without specialist training. Nevertheless, the relative protection inherent in the career niche they occupy does not protect against change.

All occupational groups in health are faced with challenges resulting from the reform of the health care systems of CEE and CIS. New management, accounting and clinical standards are being introduced, along with new norms for numbers and types of specialties. There is pressure throughout the region for staff to deliver efficacious treatments cost-effectively and in line with EU practice. Inevitably this means individual staff having to adapt what they do, abandoning outmoded or discredited procedures and taking on new work practices.

Staff see their qualifications devalued by developments in clinical and management practice and feel disadvantaged relative to new graduates. They fear seeing their skill area downgraded, and in the case of *feldshers* and other very specialised occupations face being phased out altogether. Poor management can quickly turn opportunities for change into the grounds for stress, creating tensions between and within occupational groups. Training, continuous professional development, consultation and sensitivity to gender issues can all counterbalance these insecurities but only if they genuinely prepare all staff for new job tasks and provide ongoing support in meeting the demands of a health care system in transition. In their absence all the change taking place can and does create a sense of insecurity.

There is a distinct role for unions and professional associations in negotiating an approach to reform that does not wholly compromise job security. They are obvious partners for social dialogue in any effort to ensure that staff in all health care institutions, (whatever their relationship to central government or form of ownership), benefit from change rather than being crushed by it. It is perhaps regrettable that at a time when all workers require a clear voice, doctors' associations should be seen to be pulling away from the trade union movement and addressing more sectional interests. Doctors are the least vulnerable staff group. They are also the closest to government with their professional bodies accepting increasing statutory responsibilities for licensing and accreditation. It is quite natural that their mandate should not include the needs of other occupations but it is worrying if concern for their own career niches should distract from the needs of the system as a whole. The following recommendations seek to suggest some policy directions, which would best serve the interests of all occupational groups and promote overarching job security.

International agencies and bilateral assistance programmes should:

- acknowledge that one single model of job categories and tasks will not 'fit all' health systems at all stages of their development;

- advise countries not in rapid transition (non-accession countries) against seeking to meet EU standards in the short-term and as a primary concern;

- advocate for comprehensive regulation and control of numbers entering medical and nursing training;

- promote a commitment to retraining of staff to take on new roles, rather than replacing experienced staff with new entrants to the health sector;

- work with national governments to develop and refine training programmes for new job tasks and categories, including in primary care, public health, management and information technology;

- advocate for all proposed change to be discussed with trade unions and associations and to be gender sensitive;

- encourage links between Western European and CEE/CIS associations for nursing, midwifery and other professions allied to medicine as well as between trade unions, and otherwise support the development of a professional voice for a full range of occupational groups; and

- support research into the role of professional groups in licensing and accreditation, generating case studies and guidelines on best practice.

Governments should consider:

- enforcing a *numerus clausus* approach to restrict numbers entering the health professions through private and public routes;

- formally committing themselves to retrain staff required to change the content of their job and legislating to ensure that local government and private sector employers extend similar guarantees to staff;

- working with international agencies to develop and refine training programmes for new job tasks and categories, including in primary care, public health, management and information technology;

- revising in-service training and continuing professional development programmes so that they best support staff in new roles;

- reviewing the role of *feldshers*, midwives and/or public health nurses with a view to maintaining the existing job structure for autonomous nurse practitioners;

- protecting occupational groups other than doctors by mandating employers and insurance companies that negotiate directly with doctors' associations to include representatives of all professional groups in these discussions;

- involving a full range of trade unions and professional associations in changing working practices and determining standards, and in accreditation and licensing activities;

- setting out a clear road map illustrating the scope and extent of the reforms, so that trade unions are in a position to negotiate on behalf of staff, and so that staff can understand the full implications of the changes that are being made to job content and boundaries; and

- legislating to ensure that job enlargement or enrichment leading to increased responsibility (whether clinical or management) be matched by increased remuneration, fully funding appropriate pay increases for staff directly employed by central government, and mandating such increases in decentralized employment settings.

Trade unions should:

- lobby for appropriate restrictions to numbers entering training for medical, nursing and allied professions;

- insist on an active say in the introduction of change in working practices, and in the modernization of services to improve efficiency and effectiveness, including agreeing new job tasks and categories, contributing to the development of appropriate training, and deciding how it will be provided;

- act as a key route for providing information to the workforce, securing and communicating adequate and timely details of all proposed changes to working patterns, working conditions and job descriptions;

- ensure that all reforms that affect job security are discussed at a local level (through representatives of trade unions and associations) well in advance of the introduction of any change;

- identify and approach occupational groups at particular risk from changing clinical standards and definitions, including *feldshers*, therapists and rehabilitative staff, and develop tailored support and representation to directly address their job security concerns;

- monitor the impact of changes from a gender perspective to ensure that the shifting on job boundaries does not disadvantage women workers;

- establish links with professional bodies to discuss jointly the implications of standard setting and accreditation for staff in occupational groups outside medicine and nursing;

- liase with the European trade union movement and the European Union to highlight the implications of international standard setting for the job security of staff at a local level; and

- review the job content of members on an occupation-by-occupation basis and work to ensure job enlargement and increased job tasks and responsibilities are linked with commensurate increases in pay.

SKILL REPRODUCTION SECURITY [55]   6

Creating widespread access to education and training was a significant achievement of the pre-transition societies of CEE and CIS. The region enjoyed almost universal access to basic education, enormously high literacy levels and an extensive post-secondary education infrastructure. The education and health sectors collaborated to produce (largely female) doctors, nurses, pharmacists, dentists and a range of other medical and paramedical professionals all of whom were absorbed by health care systems [56]. There were also structures in place to deliver in-service training as well as to allow staff to specialize or achieve post-graduate qualifications. Although not all the education and training was at a level that would be regarded as sufficient or desirable by today's standards it turned out qualified staff who are still able to apply their skills post-transition. These staff are now being called upon to adapt to changing circumstances and to take on new tasks and responsibilities (see job security). The pressure to gain new competences however, is unlike many of the pressures to change working practices. There has often been a focus on increasing quality and responsiveness and not just efficiency. Change is therefore more often perceived by staff as being about opportunities as well as threats.

This section looks at the issues that face new entrants to the health sector and the impact that they may have on existing staff. It reviews the potential barriers to access to continuing education and retraining and addresses the skill reproduction needs of new categories of staff. It concludes that high human capital is a positive legacy of communism but that without active lobbying by trade unions and associations these assets could be lost. In particular it suggests that workers need to secure not only equal access to training but also the chance to apply that training in a safe and well-paid environment if they are not to end up moving to other sectors or other countries, or simply falling into despair.

---

[55] The IFP-SES defines Skill Reproduction Security as widespread opportunities to gain and retain skills, through apprenticeships, employment training, etc.

[56] Some sense of the scale of production is given by the Russian Federation, where even today 10 per cent of all higher education establishments and some 15 per cent of all secondary vocational educational establishments train students to work in health (Stepanchikova *et al.*, 2001).

Existing skills and initial training:
achievements and threats

Unlike in many other areas of socio-economic security, the foundations of skill reproduction have proved reasonably durable and many staff are still able to utilize the skills they acquired before transition and to update them. The ILO–PSI survey for example found that in 11 out of 14 countries providing data, employees in all occupations were using and maintaining their skills. Even in those countries where problems were identified staff felt that they could either partially apply and maintain their skills as in Lithuania, or that at least some occupations were able to do so (Afford, 2001) [57]. This constitutes a real achievement although one marred by the considerable unevenness in training provision across the region, with some occupational groups experiencing significant barriers to access (see also below).

Preserving the skills that exist within the health sector is important. Acquiring qualifications in the first place however, is the starting point for all skill reproduction security. The availability and quality of basic education and training are crucial for the next generation of workers in the health sector.

Traditionally, recruitment into initial education programmes was based upon anticipated demand for staff, which was modelled using centrally determined norms, and in light of the skills and age profile of the workforce. Emphasis was placed on tertiary care provision and maintaining high staff to population ratios, which translated into high rates of recruitment. Since transition however there has been pressure to reduce staff and in particular to cut back on physician numbers relative to population [58]. These pressures have not, by and large, translated into significant job cuts. They have however, had an impact on the places made available through government nursing and medical schools.

Numbers of entrants (particularly to medical schools) were cut in an effort to reduce overall staff levels in the medium-term [59]. The impact of these cuts was

---

[57] In Poland clinical staff (specifically doctors and nurses) could maintain their skills while those in professions allied to medicine, support services or administration were not. Moldova, in contrast, reported that only administrative staff were maintaining their skills while all other groups were losing ground.

[58] Section 3 on Labour Market Security contains a full discussion of the assumptions underpinning international advice on staff numbers and the implications of applying these assumptions to a labour rather than capital-intensive sector.

[59] The impact of the establishment of private sector medical and nursing schools is discussed below. They did affect numbers of training places but only in some countries and not immediately on transition. Even then the students recruited did not graduate and enter the labour market for a number of years.

not felt in the first instance because of the age profile of those already employed in the sector and the widespread practice of pensioners continuing to work after retirement. Most importantly the length of medical education meant that there was no immediate impact on numbers graduating, and indeed the numbers of physicians leaving medical school actually increased in the first few years after transition. This reflected the general growth in medical school places across the region in the late 1980s. By 1995 however, the cuts had worked their way through the system and the number of new doctors being produced had fallen back to 1990 levels or below in most countries (fig. 15). [60]

The position with regard to nurses is much more mixed, so while some countries have reduced the numbers graduating others (especially those with low numbers of nurses in 1990) have seen increases in graduate production (fig. 16).

The number of (almost exclusively female) midwifery graduates is linked to the number of nurses and unsurprisingly has no clear pattern either. However, low and falling birth rates in some countries have led to rather more rapid reductions in the numbers of midwives being trained. The production of dentists (who in much of the region are a sub-set of doctors) has closely tracked the production of physicians, with an initial rise in graduates to 1995 and a subsequent decline (fig. 17). Pharmacists, the only other group for which data are available, are generally graduating in declining numbers.

Figure 15. Numbers of physicians graduating per 100'000 population, selected countries 1990, 1995 and 2000 (formal sector only)

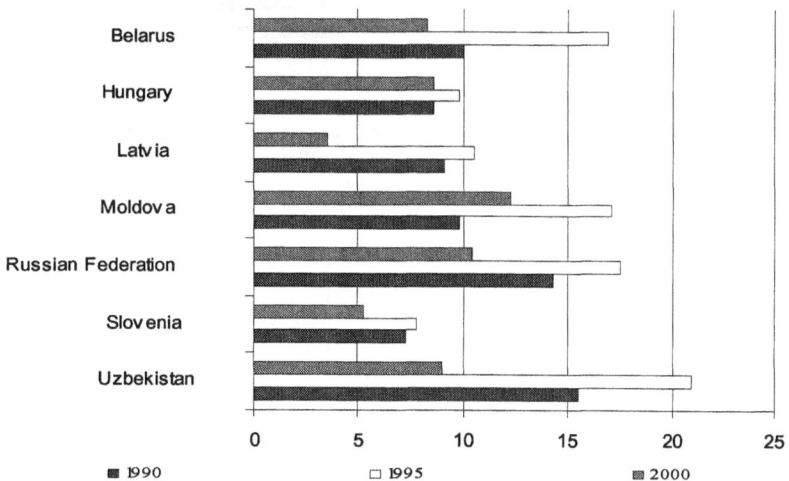

Source: (WHO, 2002b).

---

[60] Although the three following figures cover the same time period, the values on the y -axis are of a quite different scale in each case.

Figure 16. Numbers of nurses graduating per 100'000 population, selected countries 1990, 1995 and 2000 (formal sector only)

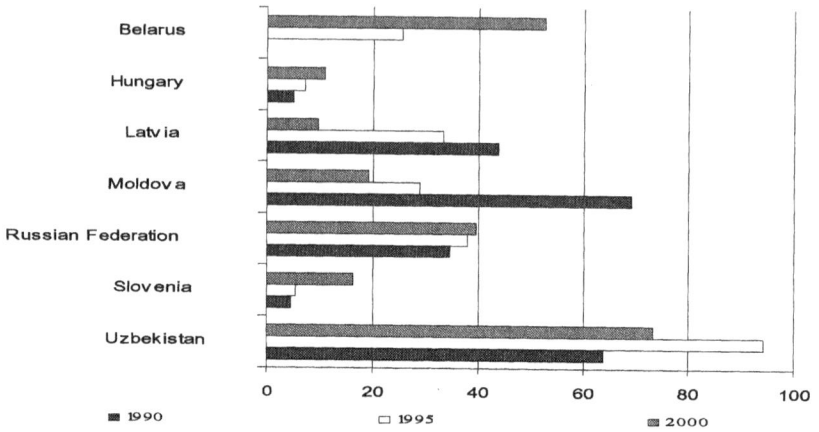

Source: (WHO, 2002b).

Figure 17. Numbers of dentists graduating per 100'000 population, selected countries 1990, 1995 and 2000 (formal sector only)

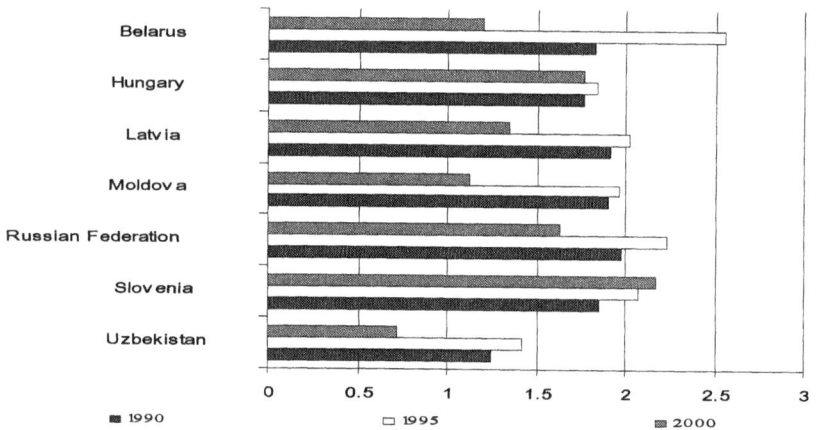

Source: (WHO, 2002b).

At the same time as public sector medical and nursing schools were cutting places, many establishments reviewed their curricula and revised the teaching offered to better reflect the needs of post-transition health care systems. There were efforts, often in partnership with international agencies, to address the importance of non-communicable disease and to better accommodate primary care and public health in undergraduate syllabuses. The formal, recognized providers of education and training for the health sector were therefore improving (or attempting to improve) the quality of graduates as they were reducing their numbers.

The effort to reduce the capacity of state training establishments in some countries has foundered however, in the face of new private medical and nursing schools. These have sprung up to meet demand from students missing out on places in the public sector and are often effectively unregulated. There are no controls on the numbers of students private institutions accept, on the criteria they use to govern admissions and no accreditation process governing their standards (although they seek to mirror state sector syllabuses). There is considerable uncertainty as to how to treat their graduates. Armenia, Georgia and the Republic of Moldova for example, are all struggling with the issue of "private qualifications" although their Ministries of Health appear to feel they have little choice but to recognize them, if only because of the investment of time and money on the part of the students concerned.

The position is obviously undesirable in terms of the individuals affected. It also bodes ill for the health system as a whole, which faces the threat of uncontrolled, overprovision of staff. It is also of course, extremely worrying for those staff already in health services. Overproduction of new entrants can only depress the labour market and undermine the bargaining power of workers.

Continuing education and training: dealing with opportunity and obsolescence

Staff from all occupational groups may feel uncertain about their future but the pressures for change (since many of them revolve around raising standards) ultimately create opportunities to use and maintain skills (except where these are obsolete) as well as gain new ones. The ability to enhance and extend competencies however depends on the availability and suitability of training or on skill reproduction security. Traditional approaches to in-service training in CEE and CIS focussed very much on doctors and involved mandated attendance on standardized courses. Career progression for physicians depended on attendance at courses triggered by the length of time spent in the job, and pay increases followed completion of the required training. The incentive for taking part was there and so staff participated but it was widely recognized that there was scope for significant improvement in the relevance and quality of the training. The provision for other occupations was less than adequate. The turmoil of transition saw many of the continuing education schemes that did exist fall into abeyance. Efforts to establish a new approach have attempted to address new job tasks and responsibilities and to take on board new professional areas [61]. The success of such approaches has been mixed.

---

[61] It is all but impossible to draw neat boundaries between different types of in-service training, continuing education and retraining. The routine updating of medical and nursing knowledge

The fact that the amount of training available to staff has increased in a number of countries is a positive sign, although availability does not necessarily imply relevance or quality. In rapid transition countries this increase in provision is often in response to the demands made by EU standards and the need to meet them, while in Croatia and Kyrgyzstan the government has passed legislation mandating training provision. The contrasting cases of Armenia, Poland and the Republic of Moldova are more worrying. A decline in the training offered may reflect simply a lack of resources, but it may also be that decentralization and privatization create confusion as to who is responsible for the design and delivery of training and who it is who has to pay for it.

It is also troubling that barriers to access are reported, sometimes even in countries where the availability of training is increasing on paper. Kyrgyzstan and the Russian Federation for example, both report difficulties of access that seem to be linked to the physical distances between staff and training provision. One of the more common blocks appears to be lack of staff time, which implies that management are not prioritising their participation in training, although staff may simply feel they cannot afford to be away from the workplace as is the case with other forms of absence (see work security). The decline in public sector childcare provision also creates difficulties in uptake, particularly for female staff. Another crucial barrier to training and retraining is cost and several country surveys highlighted the negative role of funding constraints. Latvia reported doctors having to fund their own retraining to meet primary care requirements while in Lithuania nurses have to cover the indirect costs of reskilling. If these examples prove to be in any way typical it will severely compromise security and equity as even a cursory examination of income security demonstrates conclusively that staff could not afford to pay for training and retraining, even were these an acceptable suggestion. Finally, there are cases in Georgia and the Republic of Moldova of staff having become so demotivated that they may no longer want to participate in training.

There are few data that capture the full range of training being provided, but it seems unlikely that all occupational groups have equal access. Doctors and particular groups of nurses are clearly prioritized by most governments, and efforts to establish a family physician system often dominate training agendas. Initiatives in management, financial management and information technology also receive considerable attention. However, there are groups of nurses who graduated through accelerated training routes with relatively little 16+ education. Although there is insufficient evidence to measure accurately if they are being

---

overlaps with training to follow new treatment protocols or to work safely with new equipment, pharmaceuticals or prescribing regimes. Similarly, it is not easy to say when the ordinary development of management and accounting skills constitutes retraining in finance or computing. There are career niches that are quite distinct and require very particular training (primary care or general practice, public health) but otherwise ongoing training and retraining are treated as a single continuum here.

treated in the same way as their "better" qualified colleagues or given similar access to training, there is a powerful suggestion that they are regarded as a "second tier" of nursing staff and that less is being invested in their development, creating real skill reproduction insecurity. Nor do less than glamorous nursing assignments like care of the elderly or the mentally ill attract training funds. Whether support staff, administrators or orderlies are given opportunities to enhance their skills is even less clear.

Nor is it known how the staff and skill needs created by the shift to insurance-based systems are being addressed. Many countries have introduced systems that demand contractual (or quasi-contractual) relationships between patients and insurers, the third-party purchasers of care, and between purchaser and providers. The monitoring of those contracts, the management of reimbursement systems and the pooling of risk all posit particular skills and therefore particular training. It would be interesting to know whether this training has been provided and if so who had access to it and who paid for it.

Data are also in short supply when it comes to measuring how effective the training provided actually is in helping staff meet the challenges of new roles. This is particularly true for small-scale training initiatives but is also the case where there has been significant investment on the part of governments and donors in key areas like the training of general practitioners and public health nurses, or the creation of public health and management specialists. These initiatives are of course evaluated but the evaluation tends to measure technical content or quality of delivery rather than the extent to which participants can apply the skills they acquire [62].

The ability to use training reflects not just on its design and execution but also on the work environment to which the trainees will return. Computing skills are no use, for example, without a suitable computer and a constant electricity supply. There is some evidence that cohorts of general practitioners trained in the Russian Federation were returned to work in old-style polyclinics, a setting which is not conducive to the practice of family medicine, and so reverted to previous patterns of care delivery (Tragakes et al., 2002). There is also anecdotal evidence that significant numbers of trainees on internationally sponsored management programmes exited the health sector as a result of resistance within the system to their putting into practice what they had learned. This gap between learning and its application may help to explain the discouragement reported by Georgian and Moldovan workers. It also demonstrates clearly that access to training does not guarantee skill reproduction security.

The direct implication of restructuring any health system is that, just as new skill needs emerge, some skills become obsolete. This is not the same

---

[62] Examples are available at www.worldbank.org.

phenomenon as whole jobs falling foul of EU norms [63]. It is more a case of statisticians who were adept at complex calculations finding that relatively unskilled computer operators can fulfil their tasks or of nurses who carried out programmes of child health checks finding that the approach they took is no longer regarded as evidence-based or appropriate. This is likely to be particularly relevant in countries reducing the number of job categories they recognize and shifting between models of care provision. These changes pose a powerful threat to the staff whose skills no longer match the profile of the reformed health sector. There is little to be gained however, from insisting that redundant practices are continued or that training be preserved once the occupation it relates to is superfluous. The focus should instead be ensuring that the opportunities created by development are open to precisely those staff who are threatened by obsolescence and on guaranteeing sufficient and appropriate training to equip them for new roles. This is all the more important because pension provision in most of the region is inadequate, ruling out early retirement as an acceptable option for staff nearing the end of their working lives.

Unions and associations: guarantors of security

Trade unions and professional associations have a vital role to play in addressing the gap between the demand for change and the needs and ability of staff to respond to that change. As with job security there is a need for a collective voice on the issue of numbers entering the professions, more particularly on the position of private medical and nursing school graduates. Most importantly though, unions and associations must ensure training is provided where needed and without charge, and that it meets the needs of staff, including those whose skills are most vulnerable to obsolescence. Unions and associations are also best placed to ensure that access to training is equitable in gender terms, so that a predominantly female sector does not train disproportionate numbers of men for the highest paying specialities or indeed exclude men from opportunities to enhance their skill reproduction security.

Unions and associations across the region identify training as a core concern and many, as in Bulgaria, Latvia, and Slovakia, play an active part in communicating what it is that staff need and developing a response. Others, the Czech Republic being a case in point, take no part in provision but help determine training policy and lobby for paid leave and allowances for staff under-going training. That said there are worrying instances like Croatia where unions are explicitly excluded from consultations on training and retraining (Afford, 2001). Nonetheless in general, there seems to be government recognition that there need be no conflict between the unions' concern with

---

[63] For a discussion of the impact of change on *feldshers* see Section 5, Job Security.

maintaining their members' professional status and the wider agenda of workforce development which seeks to enhance skills across the board [64].

There are potential conflicts of interest however, in cases where professional associations, and doctors' associations in particular, are given responsibility for accreditation and licensing. Essentially they must perform as advocates for the needs of their constituency while acting as guarantors of "objective" standards, thus running the risk of compromising one or other responsibility. Unions do not face these divided loyalties and are perhaps best placed to work for staff to achieve the best possible access to and design of training, which will in turn have the best possible chance of being accepted and ultimately utilized "on the shop floor" (Scrivens, 1997).

Skills, opportunity and emigration

Data are scarce but it is already clear that there is some demand in Western Europe for the recruitment of trained staff from CEE and CIS, particularly nurses. Norwegian and Italian hospitals amongst others have been reported recruiting mainly female nursing staff in CEE, sometimes to take up less responsible yet better paid positions as nursing auxiliaries. Although the scale of staff movement is still limited it is likely to become an increasingly common phenomenon as the borders of the EU move eastwards over the next decade (Jennet, 2002). There is also emerging evidence of emigration between the countries of CEE, so nurses from Slovakia have moved to the Czech Republic, which provides better conditions for staff. This mobility will be all the easier as training standards are harmonized and recognition of qualifications is under-written by the EU. It will inevitably exacerbate the current difficulties that CEE and CIS countries have in recruiting and retaining staff in rural areas [65].

This is not to suggest that the free movement of workers should be prevented. It is rather to highlight the fact that if low wages and poor working conditions in Eastern Europe persist there is likely to be a significant skills drain to the West, with the best trained and most dynamic staff being "poached" first. It is ironic that skill reproduction security will actually contribute to this and that the inputs of international donors will have helped design and deliver training that allows the East of Europe to subsidize the West.

---

[64] The fact that unions have a recognized interest in training should not disguise the fact that their role overall is significantly less extensive than in the past, see Section 8, Voice Representation Security.

[65] Brain drain to the West must be seen in light of "the induced 'internal brain drain'" which Standing identifies as a major cause for concern. Highly qualified staffs, including doctors, are already leaving the health sector in order to take up commercial opportunities that will earn them "above-subsistence" incomes within CEE and CIS. The threat of losses to the EU must be understood in this context (Standing, 1996).

Conclusions and policy recommendations

Workers in most occupations in health have traditionally had high levels of both education and training. Nevertheless, a retrospective review of curricula and qualifications in place at the time of transition does suggest that the region had fallen behind the West in terms of the content of medical and related courses and the teaching methodologies used. There was a tendency to focus on communicable disease and to undervalue responsiveness to patients. Notwithstanding these shortcomings, there was a very extensive skill reproduction infrastructure in place which continues to function. This legacy of the past is enormously valuable and worth preserving. It is not however, sufficient to provide workers with the security they need in constantly changing health systems.

The existence of training infrastructures in all the countries of the region has not in practice meant guaranteed access to training for all the groups of staff in the health sector. Some of this failure to deliver universal benefits stems from the fact that training is primarily designed for and targeted at occupations, like family physicians, that are intended to play a pivotal role in health sector reforms. This is often the case even where these groups represent only a tiny fraction of the health sector personnel and where no structures are in place to support them in applying their newly acquired skills. This preoccupation distracts attention from occupations like nursing the elderly or the mentally ill, which are almost without exception, regarded as unglamorous and are ignored in training terms.

Insecurity is also rooted in the barriers individual staff encounter in trying to access training. Some of these relate to the physical isolation of staff in rural areas, (although staff in towns and cities other than the capital also seem to have restricted options) and some to the lack of training for particular occupations mentioned above. One of the most significant blocks is money. Staff asked to cover the cost of training, or even its indirect costs are put in an impossible situation. Even when there is no charge, simply being away from work can mean an unsupportable drop in income for staff who depend on informal payments to supplement their earnings. Insecurity however is not just a matter of availability, distribution or access. There are also major questions about how good the training on offer is and, more to the point, how well it enables staff to use their skills. Theoretical or academic courses are well and good but cannot always give staff the opportunities they need to gain and retain workable competences.

Getting the balance of education and training right is an essential element in producing a workforce motivated and able to deliver high quality and responsive health care within reformed health sectors. Getting it right though can be a double-edged sword as the more skilled workers become the more likely it is that they will be targeted for recruitment by Western European employers. There is a danger implicit in raising skill and qualification levels at a time when the governments of CEE and CIS are unable to provide staff with pay and conditions, which compete with those in the West. The danger is that the investment involved will simply equip staff to move away and so will ultimately benefit richer health care systems. The following recommendations are intended to address some of the challenges of achieving skill reproduction security, despite these possible (negative) consequences of success.

International agencies and bilateral assistance programmes should:

- make a clear commitment to training for all occupational groups;

- prioritize (in their work with national governments) initiatives which address the training needs of staff other than doctors and nurses;

- advocate for national governments to secure formal trade union and association involvement in training design and delivery and insist that unions and associations are partners in any sponsored or joint training initiatives;

- lobby EU institutions to establish a levy to be paid by Western European institutions recruiting CEE or CIS trained staff, with the levy to be paid into a training and development fund in the country of origin of the recruit;

- support a survey of skills training provided to all occupational groups on a country-by-country basis with a view to identifying the provision for staff other than doctors and nurses and highlighting any regional or gender inequities; and

- sponsor a qualitative study of the impact of different training models/styles on working practices; drawing out obstacles that inhibit the application of lessons learned and factors that facilitate uptake; and generating case studies and guidelines on training design.

Governments should:

- formulate an explicit partnership agreement with national trade unions and associations to design, monitor and deliver training systems and for the development and implementation of all the recommendations below;

- provide guidelines and regulation to ensure that the standard-setting and accreditation functions of professional associations do not compromise, or are not compromised by, their role as advocates for sectional interests;

- regulate private sector medical and nursing schools appropriately and ensure that the production of staff by the private sector is factored into national human resource planning initiatives;

- establish quality criteria for training and a register of recognized training activities and/or providers for the full range of occupations in health;

- institute a certification or accreditation process for all health care institutions that includes explicit targets for the training of all staff *i.e.* all occupational groups, with the training to meet agreed quality criteria;

- ensure that all government and insurance bodies (where they exist) only deal or contract with institutions that meet the accreditation criteria with respect to training provision for all staff;

- legislate to ensure employers, whether they are private or public sector or from parallel health systems, are obliged either to provide training that meets agreed quality criteria directly or to cover the cost of equivalent training;

- work with insurance bodies (where they exist) to address the training needs of staff in the social health insurance system and develop appropriate training, quality criteria etc.;

- monitor equity of access to training including between occupations, across regions/provinces, and in gender terms; and

- review training provision in light of the impact it has on working practices on the "shop floor".

Trade unions, and where appropriate associations, should:

- play a full part in the design and accreditation of training, exploring with government ways of ensuring that unions are represented in standard-setting;

- advocate on behalf of ancillary staff to ensure their training needs are addressed;

- ensure priority is given to training and retraining staff with obsolete skills;

- seek guarantees on access to training for staff in rural areas;

- monitor training uptake by gender and so the equity of access to new skills and higher paying areas of specialization;

- push for training of those staff with responsibility for managing change;

- track any charges levied for training and lobby to secure free provision and ensure employers or governments cover the full costs of staff participation;

- measure the uptake and applicability of training and the extent to which members are able to apply lessons learned; and

- consider positioning themselves to take on the role of training provider, perhaps working in partnership with academic institutions or professional associations.

WORK SECURITY [66] 7

The well-being of health sector staff in the work place depends on the physical conditions in which they work, their exposure to risk or violence, their hours and the psycho-social stressors around them. The pre-transition economies may not have prioritized the treatment of workers in health (since they were regarded as non-productive) but they were without exception ideologically committed to proper treatment of workers and to good practice in health and safety even if in practice this commitment did not always lead to ideal conditions. Since transition however, it seems that fewer workers are injured at work, fewer fall ill as a result of work related diseases and fewer are absent on any given day. All these might be interpreted as indicators that work security has improved in the last dozen years. In reality though the picture is far more complex.

A gulf has opened up between official statistics and formal legislation on one hand and the actual working environment on the other. This section explores how the physical conditions health workers experience have changed (sometimes for the better but often for the worse), how the ability of workers' representatives to influence health and safety has weakened and how despite formal protection against accidents, unsocial hours and night work many staff find themselves with little choice but to work in extremely difficult and deteriorating conditions. It also reviews briefly the shortcomings of disability benefits and pensions, which should protect against illness at work but which have fallen in value just like maternity, severance and unemployment pay (see employment security). Finally, it focuses on the stress that workers face, and examines how stressors help account for statistics that seem impressive while undermining the whole concept of work security.

Work conditions, injury and illness: the gap between reported and real security

Not all health sector infrastructure and equipment has declined over the last decade. The "top" end of medicine in many countries has seen the purchase of

---

[66] The IFP-SES defines Work Security as protection against accidents and illness at work, through safety and health regulations, limits on working time, unsociable hours, night work for women, etc.

highly sophisticated technologies and enhanced provision for specialist and elite services.[67] Croatia, Latvia and Lithuania report improvements in safety due to the replacement of obsolete equipment (ILO, 2001). Nonetheless, the vast bulk of health care facilities in the majority of countries have suffered from significant under investment, or neglect. The Russian Federation can furnish particularly stark examples and a brief review of Russian circumstances gives a sense of just how bad working conditions in some countries can become. In 1992, 23 per cent of hospitals had no water supply; 33 per cent, no sewage system; 30 per cent, no central heating; and 60 per cent, no hot water supply (Stepantchikova *et al.*, 2001). While 1992 was a time of particular upheaval there is little evidence of marked improvement. Stepantchikova highlights the continued crisis in rural areas, which as might be expected, face particular problems. She estimates that (in 2001) of all rural Russian hospitals "58.8 per cent of them need thorough repairs, 75.8 per cent have no sewage system, 72 per cent have no water supply, and 66.4 per cent do not have central heating". The more basic health centres providing primary care and obstetric services (POS) fared even worse with 87.2 per cent having no central heating, 93.2 per cent have no water supply and 93.7 per cent have no sewage system (Stepantchikova *et al.*, 2001). The Russian Federation clearly faces immense problems but it is not unique. World Bank and WHO reports on Albania, Armenia, Belarus, the Republic of Moldova and the countries of the Caucasus and central Asia repeatedly site similar conditions, sometimes exacerbated by civil wars but more often as a consequence of long-term under investment. There need be no detailed discussion of the correlation between working conditions, accidents and illness in these cases; a lack of heating, water and sewage systems simply must constitute unacceptable working conditions.

Even where the more extreme circumstances that face so many health sector workers are not apparent, conditions can still be problematic. Certainly they are often not significantly better than they were in 1990. When the ILO/PSI four-country survey tested the notion that conditions were generally improving, it found that although over 30 per cent of Czech respondents agreed more than 40 per cent disagreed, a figure that rose to over 60 per cent in Lithuania and Ukraine (fig. 18).

[67] Countries like the Czech Republic and Hungary where GDP has recovered faster than in CIS and where the private sector is relatively developed might have been expected to have witnessed investment in high technology equipment. It is striking however, particularly given the evidence that follows, that specialist centres in countries like Belarus and the Russian Federation have also been able to secure expensive, "cutting edge" technologies.

Figure 18. Percentage of staff reporting general improvement in working conditions

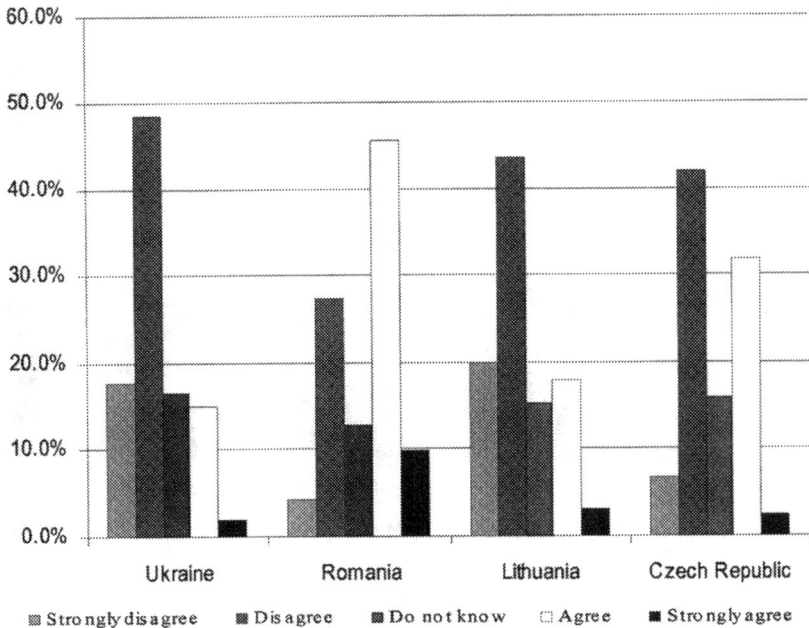

Source: (ILO, 2001).

The fact that workers did not perceive conditions as improving did not however, automatically imply that they thought conditions were getting worse. A significant number in all countries disagreed with the suggestion that the transition period (or rather the last 10 years) had seen conditions deteriorate (fig. 19). They felt similarly about the pattern of change over the last five years, although with a little less certainty about the pattern of change. That said more than 40 per cent of Lithuanian respondents and 50 per cent of those in Ukraine agreed that their working conditions had worsened in the last decade. Perhaps as telling is the number who felt that conditions in the health sector compared badly with those in other sectors or areas of industry (fig. 20). The total that perceived conditions as being poor by national standards was highest in the Ukraine at over 70 per cent, but the sense of relative disadvantage is most striking in the Czech Republic because in so many other respects Czech workers were very positive about health system conditions [68].

_____

[68] Far higher rates of respondents (over 70 per cent in all cases) disagreed with the proposition that their working conditions were excellent relative to Western standards, but this is perhaps unsurprising given the objective differences in GDP and health expenditure per capita and the widespread perception that Western Europe enjoys a high quality of life (ILO, 2001).

Figure 19. Percentage of staff agreeing that health sector working conditions had worsened over the last 10 years

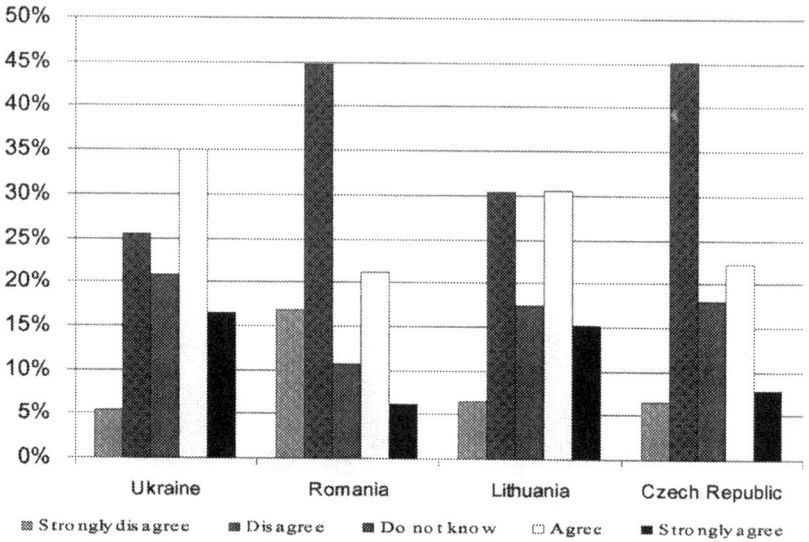

Source: (ILO, 2001).

Figure 20. Percentage of staff agreeing that health sector working conditions were excellent by national standards

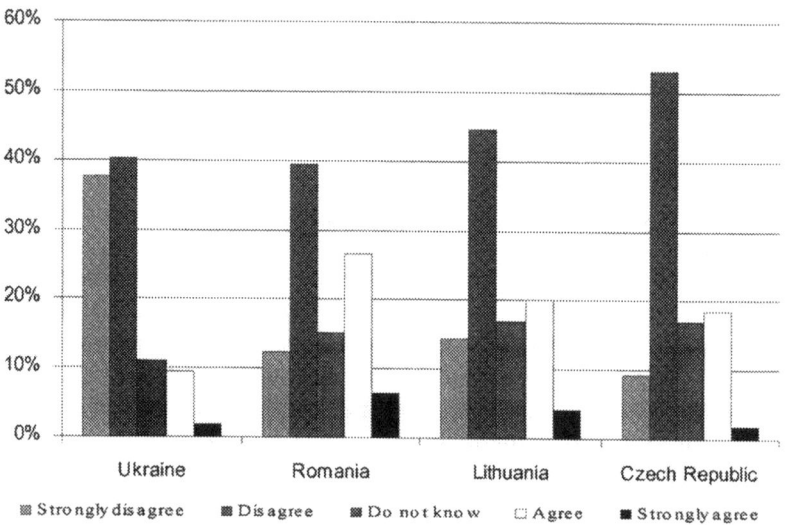

Source: (ILO, 2001).

Health sector conditions alone cannot determine work security but they do dictate the environment in which workers must spend significant amounts of time (see below)[69]. Working conditions will impact on rates of occupational injury and on the likelihood of staff acquiring a work-related illness. In the health sector there are particular risks associated with lifting and with exposure to infection, biological and chemical hazards and ionising radiation. The poor conditions that persist in CEE and CIS and the inadequacies of the infrastructure inevitably increase these risks and detract from staff security and well-being.

It might be expected that given the poor conditions reported by many, if not all health sector staff, there would have been no change or an increase in the number of accidents and injuries. However, quite the reverse is true. Not one country included in the ILO/PSI survey reported any growth in work-related injuries and Armenia, Belarus, the Czech Republic, Georgia, Kyrgyzstan, Latvia, Poland, the Russian Federation, Slovakia and Ukraine all reported a reduction in injury numbers (Afford, 2001). Often the drop was quite dramatic as in Kyrgyzstan where by 1999 the number of injuries stood at only a quarter of 1990 levels. Data is less complete for the number of days work lost to injury, but similar falls were observed and again these were often quite marked, for example in Latvia where days of absence resulting from injury fell by 80 per cent. Although, the picture is not universal (Georgia reported a slight increase in absence due to injury and the Czech Republic saw longer average absences per injury), it is clear that fewer injuries have been reported and less sickness leave taken as a result of injuries since transition.

These data suggest there was an objective improvement in work security across CEE and CIS, rather than (or regardless of) the ongoing problems in terms of conditions described above and the challenges to the regulation of conditions described below. This strains credibility. It seems much more likely that most of the fall in the number of injuries related to changes in reporting, perhaps prompted by management reluctance to acknowledge liability. Employers may be overtly resistant to taking responsibility for injury at work or they may be conveying tacit messages that workers should not report incidents, perhaps because of concerns about the costs of compensation or insurance coverage. Underreporting must also reflect the relative weakness of staff and unions, who were poorly placed to insist on comprehensive recording of accidents and could no longer access the reporting channels (or guaranteed benefits) that had existed in the communist era. The drop in injury related absence might also reflect anxiety on the part of workers who were often too insecure, both in terms of employment and income, to report injury or to take sickness leave (see also evidence on absenteeism and "presenteeism"). The fears that inhibited workers from reporting accidents or taking time off to recover are explored more fully below but must be seen as explanatory of at least some of

---

[69] National legislation (for example on unsocial hours) or the degree of societal tension (which will contribute to levels of violence) can serve as examples of the "external factors" that help determine work security.

the nominal improvement in injury rates.[70] They strongly suggest a more insecure not a safer environment.

There are very few reliable data available on work-related disease and the working days lost as a result of it. The data that do exist tend to suggest less cases of disease and less absence as a result of disease (except in the Republic of Moldova, which saw a slight increase in illness related absence between 1990 and 1991). Again there is the probability that reluctance on the part of staff to report illness and to take sickness leave that will mean being away from the workplace (and from the source of direct payments) is artificially depressing the levels of the problems that exist. Certainly detailed data from Russia point to an increase in "occupational incidents" among health care workers (table 8), evidence borne out by reports of increased cases of tuberculosis, hepatitis, asthma and allergies amongst health sector staff Stepantchikova *et al.*, 2001).

Table 8.   Index of occupational incidents among health care workers compared with the industry average, 1990–1999

Year	Number of cases for medical workers	Index per 10'000 health care workers	Industry average index per 10'000 workers
1990	161	0.49	1.96
1991	135	0.25	2.08
1992	134	0.59	1.88
1993	209	0.67	1.85
1994	205	0.57	1.81
1995	261	0.71	1.89
1996	267	0.74	2.33
1997	318	0.88	2.32
1998	415	1.66	1.85
1999	434	1.74	1.77

Source: (Stepantchikova *et al.*, 2001).

Although it is not entirely clear how the boundaries of incidents are defined *vis-à-vis* injuries and disease the picture of increasing numbers of cases in absolute terms and per 10'000 health care workers demonstrates that there was a significant increase in risk for workers in Russia between 1990 and 1999. Most disturbingly the index for the rate of incidents, which had been significantly lower than in industry as a whole, was on a par with industry levels by 1999 (fig. 21).

---

[70] Anecdotal evidence from a number of countries suggests injuries were over-reported before 1990 and that it was part of custom and practice for staff to take sickness leave up to an informal norm. Greater insecurity would explain the ending of this practice and some of the drop in injuries and days of work lost as a result.

Figure 21. Incidence of occupational incidents for health care workers compared to industry figures 1990–1999

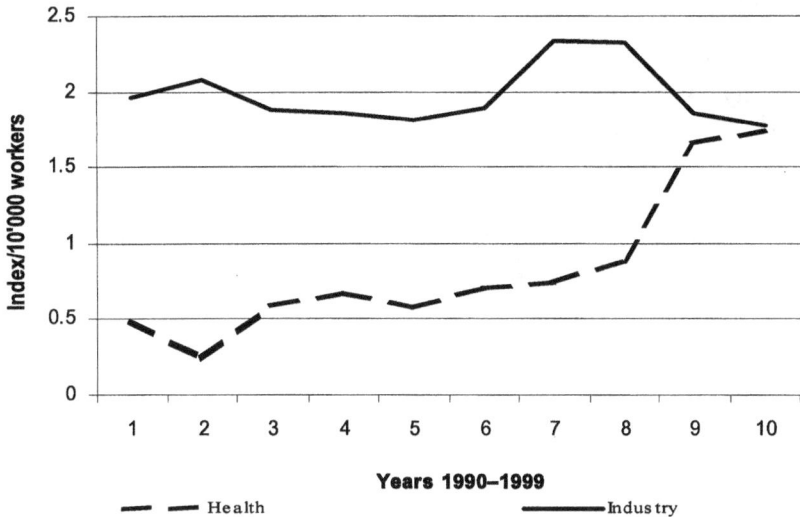

Source: Based on data supplied by Stepantchikova *et al.*, 2001.

Stepantchikova *et al* (2001) attributes the increase in disease in health care staff in the Russian Federation directly to worsening working conditions but also points out that cases of disease are more frequent among "workers with less than five years of service". This may overstate the importance of the transmission of infection at work and underplay the importance of the rising incidence of tuberculosis, hepatitis (B and C), HIV/AIDs, and other sexually transmitted infections in the wider population. Certainly the Russian Federation, like much of the region, is experiencing a sharp increase in the levels of a number of communicable diseases (often linked to poverty, poor living conditions and nutrition, high degrees of stress and diminished access to health care provision) and health care workers are not immune to these wider trends. Nonetheless, if new workers are more likely to get ill this may suggest that lack of experience and inadequate training have contributed to their acquiring infections at work [71]. Any evidence of health system failures increasing employees' exposure to risk is worrying, not least because of the life threatening nature of the infections concerned. Most infections, and certainly HIV/AIDs, ought not to pose any threat to staff in a properly regulated environment since workplace transmission is avoidable if proper procedures are followed. If suitable training and supervision are not in place and less experienced staff are more vulnerable to infection this bodes ill for employees and health system users alike.

---

[71] There may be a higher prevalence of communicable diseases in younger people and this, rather than exposure to infection in the workplace, could account for the raised risk of infection in new staff.

It is not possible to extrapolate directly from the Russian case to the rest of CEE or CIS, but the Russian experience is worth bearing in mind in reviewing the credibility of data on work-related disease across the region. Like Russia, many countries have difficult working conditions, increasingly unhealthy populations and report a lack of resources for training (see skill reproduction security) or for measures to protect health care system staff and, as in Russia, work security may be threatened by occupational exposure to infection. The fact that this insecurity is not captured by the data does not mean it does not exist.

Absenteeism — presenteeism — hours worked: evidence of insecurity

Absenteeism is falling in the health sectors of CEE and CIS. This reflects the decrease in days lost to injury or disease, and also captures a reduction in annual leave, compassionate leave, and unexplained or occasional absences from work. Most importantly of all it reveals an enormous reluctance on the part of workers to be away from work. Over and over again the ILO/PSI survey found that fear of dismissal and concern about the loss of income that would follow from any absence were seen as reasons for declining rates of absence. Decreases in numbers of injuries or the incidence of work-related disease or general increases in population health were never offered as explanations of the "improvements" seen on paper [72].

Many workers are clearly under considerable financial pressure to go to work rather than taking any type of leave of absence. This is in part because benefit levels in some countries, Poland for example, fall below standard rates of pay and in part because some employers refuse to pay staff for the full annual leave entitlement [73]. It is also and importantly, because being away from the workplace rules out access to over-time or performance related bonuses, and to under-the-table payments. In fact, the pressures on staff are so strong that in all the countries surveyed except the Czech Republic, Russian Federation and Ukraine, workers were reported as attending work when ill or when they were entitled to some other form of leave. This phenomenon, known as presenteeism suggests that work security is tenuous at best (table 9).

---

[72] Any claim that falling absenteeism could be explained by improvements in population health would be laughable in the face of overwhelming evidence of increased morbidity (including chronic and psycho-social conditions) and mortality across the region (WHO, 2002b).

[73] Staff in the Russian Federation are entitled to a basic 24 days leave rising to between 30 and 48 days depending on qualifications, years of service and exposure to harmful conditions or stress (staff in psychiatry, infectious diseases or radiology typically having increased entitlement). In practice however, many medical institutions do not provide holidays for workers, despite their legal rights, because of a lack of funds (Stepantchikova *et al.*, 2001).

Table 9. **Reasons given for staff going to work when they might be absent**

Armenia	Real income derives only from payments by patients, absence from work reduces earnings.
Kyrgyzstan	Financial motivation.
Lituania	Employees are afraid to lose job and to earn less.
Republic of Moldova	Financial needs

Source: (Afford, 2001).

Data from the WHO (fig. 22) show that the absenteeism trend across economies as a whole is much more mixed. This suggests that health sector staff experience particular insecurity and are more subject to presenteeism than in other sectors.

Figure 22. Absenteeism from work due to illness by country, 1990–1999

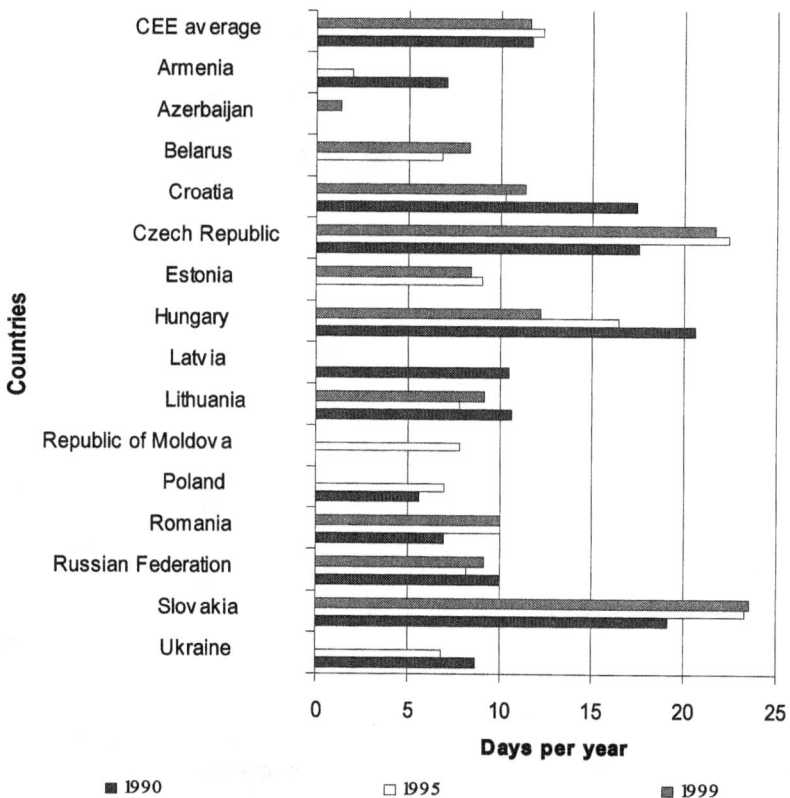

Source: (WHO, 2002b).

Not only do health sector staff work when they might be on leave. They also work long hours, frequently do overtime and often hold more than one job (see labour market security) [74]. The four-country survey demonstrates that this is not generally regarded as a problem with more than 60 per cent of respondents in each country claiming to be happy with their hours (fig. 23). Nonetheless, the satisfaction staff derive from work, its sustainability, and its safety, are inextricably linked with the number of hours worked. Excessive hours, even when they are entered into voluntarily, inevitably undermine the balance between work and home life and have often been linked with increased stress, higher levels of smoking and alcohol use and a raised risk of accidental injury [75].

Figure 23. Percentage of staff happy with the (current) hours worked

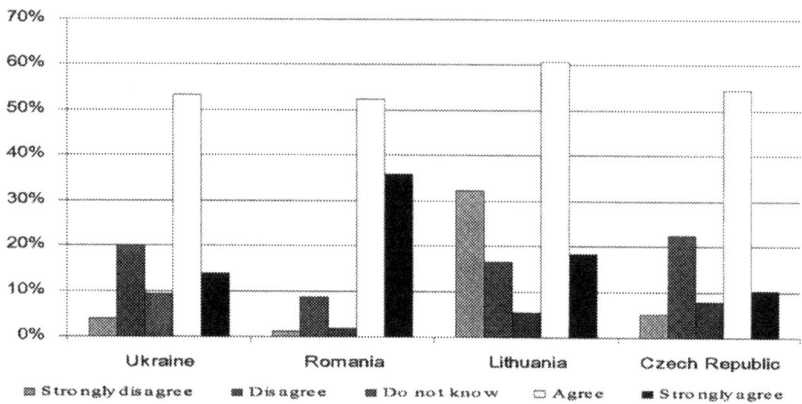

Source: (ILO, 2001).

The reason staff have often opted to work long hours without complaint or that they take on multiple jobs is that they prioritized additional income over safe limits to working time. In the Czech Republic, for example, where the adoption of a Labour Code on working hours constrained overtime, it appears that job vacancies were deliberately left unfilled and the tasks redistributed between remaining staff in order to circumvent the directive and allow for extra payments to be made (ILO, 2001). The Czech example indicates collusion between management and staff. This is not always the case. In Ukraine there is anecdotal evidence that staff have been obliged to work additional shifts and take on extra responsibilities but are not remunerated for these in any way. It

---

[74] In the Russian Federation around half of health sector workers combined their formal roles with additional work, while about a third did so in Belarus, Bulgaria and Moldova (ILO, 2001).

[75] Some of the analysis of the high morbidity and mortality levels tends to blame the victims of smoking and alcohol or drug use, suggesting that individuals are engaging in (culturally bounded) destructive behaviours. It is important to see these behaviours, however ill advised, in the context of the stressors faced by workers and to understand them as part of a gamut of coping strategies.

seems they are too scared of losing their jobs to refuse and that the satisfaction they express with their working hours must be interpreted with caution.

Whether the additional hours worked by health sector staff are taken on by choice and in exchange for extra pay or because of coercion and without recompense, a 60-hour working week is not conducive to the health or well-being of workers [76].

Legislative protection: enforcing health and safety

Staff should be protected from long and anti-social hours by health and safety legislation, just as they should be protected from harmful conditions and exposure to hazards. The centrally planned economies provided legal guarantees on a full range of health and safety issues and much of this formal protection is still in place, which should strike a positive note. The reality of work in health systems however, suggests that while the regulations are still good, they are often no longer enforced. Problems have stemmed in part from a lack of resources to update equipment and maintain adequate working conditions [77]. They also reflect the difficulties trade unions have encountered in trying to influence management decisions in increasingly decentralized health systems (see also voice representation security).

A case in point is the role of trade unions in Health and Safety Committees. In virtually all the countries of the region hospital managers are still mandated by law to involve unions in these committees or in other joint labour-management efforts. Many unions however, find themselves excluded. In Armenia as few as 10 per cent of hospitals actually allowed union representatives to participate. In other countries (although not all), the compulsory inspections designed to prevent facilities flouting potentially life-saving regulations have fallen into abeyance or been discontinued by employers [78]. This leads all too often to hit and miss implementation of rules and haphazard application of penalties for employers who breach the laws that still exist.

The situation would no doubt improve with suitable equipment and training and the wherewithal to implement good hygiene standards or if some of the powers of trade unions and health and safety committees were reinstated.

[76] Doctors and nurses in Latvia and Ukraine routinely work an average of 60 hours, while doctors in Poland may work up to 90 hours a week (ILO, 2001).

[77] Difficulties in maintaining safety were reported to be a direct result of worsening working conditions in Armenia, Poland, the Republic of Moldova, and Slovakia (ILO, 2001).

[78] The Czech Republic makes an interesting exception. The execution of safety measures is regarded as exclusively an employer's competence yet trade unions exert real influence through their delegated powers of inspection and through their expert inputs into draft legislation.

However, safety measures cannot be expected to hold up where there is insufficient funding, and where the workers' representatives most likely to champion them, are excluded or discouraged from involvement.

Benefits and pensions: no longer underwriting security

Sickness, invalidity and disability benefits all contribute to work security because they allow staff who are injured or made ill by work to take the time they need to recover (Standing, 1996, p. 227). On paper, benefits have remained unchanged. In 1999 replacement rates were generally relatively generous and although they varied from country to country, the typical range was from 80 to 100 per cent of normal pay. Countries like Croatia, with benefit as low as 10 per cent of the average wage, were very much the exception rather than the rule. The positive impression was reinforced by the fact that few barriers to access were reported and that the duration of the benefits was good, lasting effectively as long as the illness or until disability was verified [79, 80]. Nevertheless, problems do exist, not least because of the enormous erosion in the value of cash benefits and the loss of access to benefits in-kind (see employment security). The evidence on presenteeism illustrates clearly that the benefits available are simply not sufficient to afford staff real security.

Old age pensions are a more complex case, as they were traditionally a grey area of socio-economic life in Eastern Europe, reflecting some ambivalence about retirement from employment. Retirement pensions typically paid low cash amounts, in part because it was assumed that non-cash benefits would provide for the needs of the retired *äthis* in line with Leninist thinking about the "decommodification of labour" (Standing, 1997, p. 1344). However, the in-kind and social benefits that were available were often not substantial enough to offset the low-income levels provided by the state. This "shortfall" of income in combination with the relatively early entitlement to pensions, led to high levels of "working pensioners" in CEE and CIS, and to a widespread expectation that pensioners would continue to work well into retirement.

The post-communist governments of Eastern Europe have sought to reduce the numbers of retirees in work and to reform the overall pattern of retirement in response to the costs of the system and international pressures to reduce benefits

---

[79] There is not enough information to assess the impact of temporary or commercial contracts on eligibility for benefits, but the casualization of work is likely to undermine the entitlements of non-permanent staff in the longer-term.

[80] Although as Standing makes clear "often, the disability pension has been made conditional on non-receipt of unemployment benefit" (Standing, 1996, p. 241).

(Standing, 1996, pp. 229–231, 239–241) [81]. Reforms generally tried to raise the state retirement age and to make pension payments more realistic as a sole source of income. This was intended both to ease financial pressures on governments and to enhance the position of genuine retirees (raising pension-derived income and ending delays to payments). However such policies have had mixed results, and in some countries pension levels have remained below the poverty line [82]. As a consequence pensioners still play an active role in the labour market, albeit that in some countries this is less and less common (table 10) [83, 84].

Table 10. Pensioners in work, selected countries, 1990 and 1999

	Percentage of staff who were pensioners 1990	Percentage of staff who were pensioners 1999
Belarus	10	15
Bulgaria	20	2
Georgia	36	28
Kyrgyzstan	32	18
Lithuania	22	12
Poland	2	6
Russian Federation	—	40

Source: (Afford, 2001).

Again, the lesson here is that data suggesting a reasonable level of work security must be treated with a certain amount of scepticism. Good entitlement to pensions does exist but the amounts of support available are often too low to fulfil their intended purpose Quality of working life and work security depend not only on the physical conditions staff experience, (the nature of the risks they are exposed to, the hours they work), but also on the psycho-social stresses around them. All health sector staff inevitably experience real and considerable stress as a direct consequence of the type of work they do. The death of patients, contact with bereaved families and involvement in cases of childhood illness or disability are inherently stressful and will affect workers whatever country they

[81] Despite crises in health status in CEE and CIS, life expectancy has increased over the last few decades such that it has become financially untenable for governments to routinely pay the "working retired" twice, (once as wages and once as pension).

[82] In Russia for example, pension income for medical workers has got worse since 1991. Most disturbingly particular groups have fallen foul of changes in what constitutes a "legal entity" so workers in clinics and medical research organizations, doctors-statisticians, hospice directors, chief medical nurses and dietetic nurses are no longer entitled to any retirement pensions at all (Stepantchikova *et al.*, 2001).

[83] For full account of pension reform see Standing (1996, pp. 240–41).

[84] For full account of the situation in Ukraine and Russia see Standing (1997, p. 1350).

are in and regardless of whether they function in a planned or market economy. What is striking however, is how many stressors in CEE and CIS stem directly from the difficulties of life in transition economies [85].

The ILO/PSI survey identified pressures linked to particular national circumstances like the war in Croatia or privatization in Poland and stemming from particular instances of hardship, for example a shortage of medicines in Bulgaria. Bad working conditions were also mentioned, as was the impact of worsening health within a country. Overwhelmingly though the problems highlighted were associated with economic conditions and the threat of job losses (Afford, 2001). Staff repeatedly identified inadequate pay, delays in receiving wages and the fear of losing their income source altogether as the root causes of stress (table 11).

Table 11. Causes of stress, selected countries

Armenia	1. Threat of being laid off, transition to a contract system.
	2. Arrears in wages.
	3. Insolvency of the majority of patients.
Bulgaria	1. Bad working conditions.
	2. Crisis in medical institutions, absence of medicines.
Croatia	1. War situation (1990–1995).
	2. Fear of dismissal.
Lithuania	1. Fear of losing job.
	2. Fear of reduced or unpaid wages.
	3. Economic situation in the country and anxiety caused by wish to provide services of good quality.
Republic of Moldova	1. No guarantees of work.
	2. Poverty and impossibility to support a family.
	3. Uncertainty about the future.
Russian Federation	1. Low income.
	2. High communal payments.
	3. Social instability.
Ukraine	1. Sudden death of a patient.
	2. Unexpected dismissal due to staff reduction.
	3. Deception.

Source: (Afford, 2001).

---

[85] Levels of stress were not necessarily believed to have increased over recent years but they were consistently felt to be high across the region (ILO, 2001).

Workers have an incredibly low locus of control over the conditions that affect them, which is stressful in itself. They cannot improve their physical environment, choose the shifts they work or rely on the benefits they are entitled to, nor are their unions able to protect them. They are increasingly at risk of violence in the work place whether through physical force (from patients or even colleagues in distress) or more frequently from psychological threats, bullying and harassment (often linked to the constant strain of reforms and downsizing) [86]. They have little choice but to work in deteriorating conditions and with little information about their futures (Tomev *et al.*, forthcoming). What is more they are tacitly obliged to subscribe to the under-reporting of injuries and illness, to forego leave entitlement and accept unsocial hours. It is ironic that the stress they are under not only denies them work security but also accounts for so many of the impressive statistics that distort the official picture of work security and disguise the very fact that a problem exists.

Conclusions and policy recommendations

Yet again there is a clear divergence between the security "enjoyed" by staff on paper and the reality they experience. Officially, the incidence of injuries at work and work-related diseases are in decline throughout the region and falling absenteeism seems to bear out the "improvement". Formal provision of disability and invalidity benefits (and to some extent pensions) seems generally to be standing up well over time. In fact many staff are just too insecure to take leave of absence, whether they are ill or owed annual leave. They work long hours and face enormous stress, not merely due to the normal strains of working in health, but instead because they do not earn enough to feel secure and are afraid of losing their jobs. What is more, many live with the expectation that things are going to get worse rather than better (see job security) [87].

Some of this insecurity is associated with the deteriorating physical environment that many workers operate in, the upshot of a lack of investment in health sector infrastructure. Some stems from the re-emergence of infectious diseases, including tuberculosis, hepatitis and HIV/AIDs, which increases

---

[86] The general definition of workplace violence in the ILO/ICN/WHO/PSI "Framework Guidelines for Addressing Workplace Violence in the Health Sector 2002" (and as adapted from the European Commission) is "Incidents where staff are abused, threatened or assaulted in circumstances related to their work, including commuting to and from work, involving an explicit or implicit challenge to their safety, well-being or health". The report highlights the risks health sector workers face in dealing with the public at times of stress and as a result of working antisocial hours, often in isolation and with access to drugs, syringes and valuable equipment. It also flags up the link between workplace pressure and bullying.

[87] Over 60 per cent of Romanian and Lithuanian respondents expected future restructuring might further erode their working conditions, while 69.0 per cent of Lithuanian, and between 30 and 40 per cent of Czech, Romanian and Ukrainian respondents, felt that future government plans would make their situation worse (ILO, 2001).

workload, brings staff into contact with stressful situations and exposes them to risk. There is also insecurity as a result of more general economic challenges that undermine benefit levels. However, the threats to work security that affect workers are not primarily about money. They are about the break down of regulation in practice. Responsibilities have been decentralized to local government and to institutions, faster than it has proved possible to create appropriate administrative structures or to train officials to maintain proper oversight. The authority of trade unions to insist that health and safety legislation is implemented has been compromised and there is no evidence that governments themselves prioritize the enforcement of safe working practices.

The poorly functioning regulatory framework translates into health sector staff working under extremely difficult conditions, and sometimes with the threat of violence. The policy-making debate however, is rarely about how to improve the basic infrastructure or enhance government supervision. Instead physicians lobby for the purchase of highly sophisticated equipment; supported by Western European manufacturers while international pressures are brought to bear for deregulation and the withdrawal of government. Neither of these strategies is designed to (or can) address the vulnerability of staff. The following recommendations seek to provide a counterbalance to these pressures and to enhance work security.

International agencies and bilateral assistance programmes should:

- recognize explicitly the role of government regulation in guaranteeing work security;

- address the underdevelopment of rural health services and promote strategies for investment in basic rural infrastructures;

- promote a review of infrastructure and conditions in parallel health services;

- insist, through conditions attached to loans and donations, that investment in infrastructure development meets basic needs and is aimed at providing appropriate technologies and not in high-technology gadgetry;

- encourage the routine involvement of trade unions and professional associations in developing, monitoring and enforcing health and safety legislation;

- support research into the underreporting of injuries and disease; and

- sponsor a review of the operation and enforcement of labour codes in Western and Eastern Europe to identify what protection is provided and evaluate the approaches in place.

Governments should be encouraged to:

- invest in the basic infrastructure of rural health services;

- restate or reinforce health and safety legislation providing for a formal role for trade unions in health and safety committees;

- insist on routine health and safety inspections and include within the remit of the inspectors responsibility for monitoring trade union involvement;

- devolve to the health and safety inspectorate the right to collect fines for non-compliance with legislation and provide an appropriate framework for enforcement;

- put in place legislation which would protect "whistleblowers" and secure the rights of workers drawing attention to breaches in health and safety policy;

- put in place mechanisms, involving trade unions, for the monitoring and recording of workplace injuries, stress related diseases and physical and psychological violence;

- formally devolve responsibility for training for all new entrants in healthy working practices to the level of the institution;

- promote workplace based measures to reduce stress and violence and to support staff experiencing them;

- provide all appropriate vaccination for staff likely to be exposed to blood products: and

- review and enhance benefit levels.

Trade unions should:

- encourage workplace representatives to compile a record of all injuries and accidents, indicating which if any were formally acknowledged;

- support "whistleblowers" calling attention to health and safety failures;

- establish mechanisms at the branch level to monitor the infringement of entitlements to leave (for holidays and during illness);

- survey members to better understand the extent and causes of presenteeism;

- insist on representation on health and safety committees and in the formal certification of compliance with legislation;

- develop and deliver training in health and safety for local staff, including in understanding and applying legislation and monitoring and recording breaches of regulations;

- consult across the region and with international counterparts to identify the most appropriate preventive measures and range of vaccinations to be provided to staff and promote best practice in terms of health protection;

- lobby government and employers to recognize the ILO definition of violence and to incorporate the reduction or elimination of violence in the health sector into health and safety policy and organizational development plans;

- campaign at a national and local level to create an awareness of the issues surrounding violence, to foster a culture which rejects physical and psychological abuse, and to establish organizational, environmental and individual-based interventions to identify and remedy it when it occurs; and

- protest all occasions where employers put the purchase of high technology before securing basic safety.

Voice Representation Security [88]

8

Depending on the views of the protagonist it is possible to argue that trade unions of the communist era gave workers a collective voice and played a significant role in shaping employment policy or to insist that unions were wholly compromised by the state and had no power independent of it. Whichever view prevails, there can be no argument but that trade unions since transition have faced a series of powerful challenges. The move to the "market" transformed their role as formal partners in social dialogue and ended their automatic economic and political incorporation into the state. The reform of health sectors across the region changed radically the environment in which they operated. The certainties of a highly structured, central planning process with clear human resource norms and incremental approaches to change, have given way to fragmentation, inconsistency and, on occasion, chaos. Even within the union sector there have been huge upheavals with a dramatic decline in membership in many countries and in union income, the emergence of new unions and the burgeoning of professional associations pursuing the demands of particular occupational groups [89].

This section reviews falling membership and the attitudes that have led many workers to leave their union. It examines what has happened to the traditional role of trade unions in protecting socio-economic security and the new groups now aspiring to act as a collective professional voice for one or other occupation. It considers how this affects voice representation security as a whole, particularly in the face of decentralization, the introduction of insurance mechanisms and privatization. It goes on to explore the hostility of some international agencies to tripartite approaches to restructuring and concludes that while the trade union movement is sorely needed there are no guarantees that it will be able to play a part in shaping health systems so that they address workers' well-being and patients' health as well as efficient service delivery.

---

[88] The IFP-SES defines Voice Representation Security as protection of a collective voice in the labour market, through independent trade unions and employer associations incorporated economically and politically into the state, with the right to strike, etc.

[89] It is still too early to identify a pattern of development as regards employers' associations and so their contribution to voice representation security is only touched on briefly in this section.

Falling membership: challenges to union strength

Trade union membership of almost 100 per cent was normal in most CEE and CIS health sectors before 1990. These figures were "inflated" as a function of the communist system and reflected societal norms rather than active union participation. It was only to be expected therefore, that transition would bring with it some significant adjustment or normalization in membership levels and the fall in some countries has indeed been quite precipitous. By 2000 membership had dropped to approximately 30 per cent in Armenia and the Czech Republic and to just 20 per cent in Lithuania and Poland[90]. More Lithuanian and Ukrainian respondents reported working in organizations without an active trade union than reported working in organizations that had a union in place (ILO, 2001), and as worryingly some 20 per cent of Ukrainian and over 30 per cent of Czech and Lithuanian respondents just did not know whether their organization had an active union or not (fig. 24). Not all countries saw such significant drops of course, and many of the countries in the ILO/PSI survey had membership levels of between 50 and 80 per cent. In many respects too, union membership in the health sector held up better than in other parts of the public sector or than in the private sector. Nonetheless all countries experienced falling membership with only Georgia, Kyrgyzstan and Ukraine claiming to have maintained membership levels above 90 per cent[91, 92].

While the fall in membership was not uniform, it was striking. Undoubtedly it was due in part to a reaction to transition itself and a rejection of the structures and organizations that were associated with "the old days". There may also be an element of the decline that is attributable to employers' and governmental attitudes. It is certainly the case that in some of the countries of the region (most notably Latvia) unions were regarded with a degree of hostility on the part of management and that in general the private sector tended to discourage union membership[93]. However for most countries management sentiments towards union membership could best be described as neutral or ambivalent (Afford, 2001). They cannot explain the scale of the change that took place.

---

[90] The rate of membership in Poland was already comparatively low in 1990, standing at 40 per cent, whereas in Lithuania the drop in membership was from 100 per cent (Afford, 2001)

[91] The validity of these data has been questioned and Figure 23 does challenge the position in Ukraine.

[92] For full details of changes in countries in the ILO/PSI survey see annexes to Afford (2001).

[93] The private sector accounted for only a small proportion of employment in the region so its affect on union membership levels should not be overstated.

Figure 24. Percentage of respondents who believed their organization had an active union

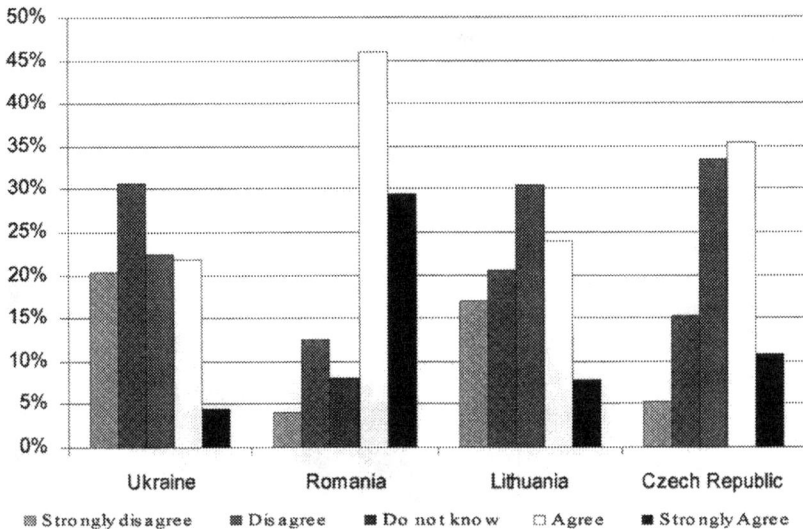

Source: (ILO, 2001).

A more depressing explanation may be provided by the attitudes of workers towards their trade unions. It seems that health sector staff increasingly feel that unions are no longer able to defend their working conditions. The views of Russian staff (where the ILO/PSI survey records union membership of 80.3 per cent) make for particularly disheartening reading. Stepantchikova reports that many union members "believe that apart from the distribution of material comforts, which are limited by budget constraints, the unions do not have the right to interfere in anything" (Stepantchikova et al., 2001). She adds that "workers also distrust their unions on the grounds that they are totally dependent on the employer's will, and, consequently, unable to protect their members in case of conflict". She also suggests collective agreements are seen as mere formalities, which for the most part have no bearing on the way workers are actually treated [94]. This bleak picture is echoed by data from elsewhere in the region. Over 40 per cent of Lithuanian and 50 per cent of Ukrainian respondents in the ILO/PSI four-country survey disagreed with the proposition that their union had been effective in protecting working conditions and, except in Romania, no more than 20 per cent of respondents actively agreed with the suggestion (fig. 25). Similarly, when asked if they believed the union had helped

---

[94] The views of Russian workers are in marked contrast to those of the Ministry of Health Care, which reported that the union and in particular the Presidium of the Central Committee of the union was working increasingly closely and effectively with the Board of the Ministry in decision-making on remuneration, benefits, labour protection and other key areas (Stepantchikova et al., 2001).

keep their jobs safe only Romanian respondents concurred in any numbers (fig. 26). Most other respondents disagreed or did not know [95].

Figure 25. Percentage of respondents who felt their union had been successful in defending working conditions

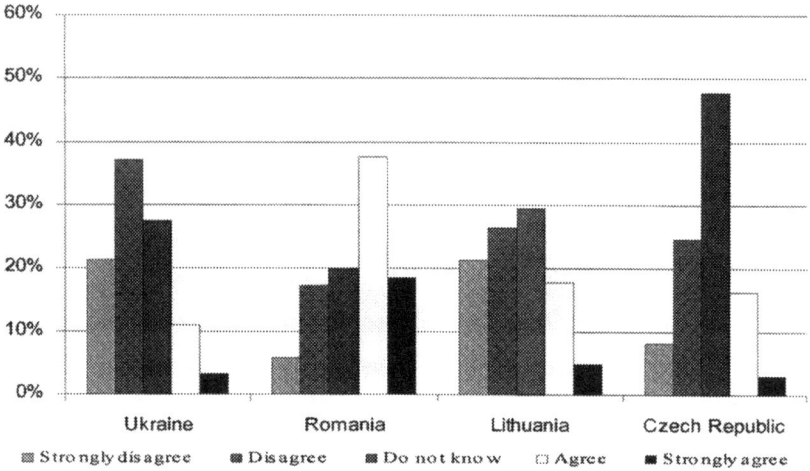

Source: (ILO, 2001).

Figure 26. Percentage of respondents who felt the union had helped keep their job safe

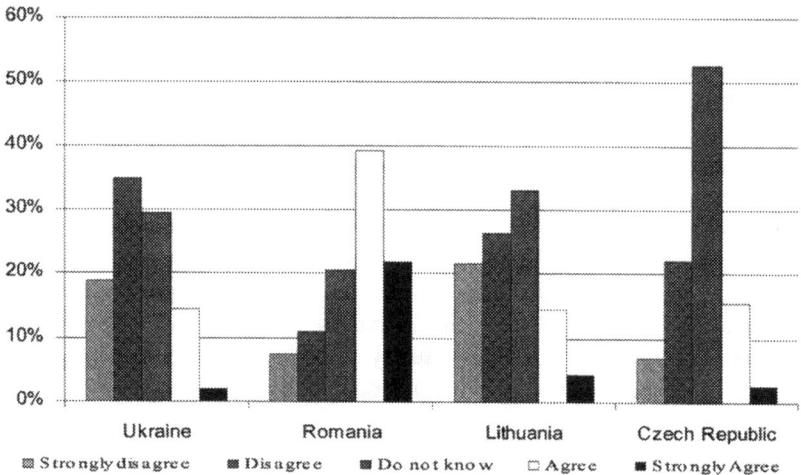

Source: (ILO, 2001).

---

[95] More respondents believed that their union had fought for their working conditions but even so responses (except in the case of Romania) were muted with only 22.1–27.4 per cent agreeing

The perceived failure of unions to protect workers and the belief that they had generally become less powerful are not the sole causes of the decline in membership, but they do play a part in discouraging participation [96]. This discouragement leads to dwindling numbers of active members, which will tend, in turn, to weaken the position of unions *vis-à-vis* management.

Union shortcomings are often not the "fault" of the unions themselves. Although some still have regular meetings with health authorities and are the strongest, if not the only voice raised on behalf of workers, most do not have the authority or the resources they need to secure results. Many are struggling to operate in an immensely complex environment and at a time of increasing resource pressure and external interference. All have severely restricted (and falling) income and many have had to make staff redundant. They can ill afford to buy in the new skills needed to respond to legislative challenges or to model the implications of reform proposals and some even have to rely on union officials working on a voluntary basis. This inevitably undermines their ability to represent staff effectively, which in turn enforces the scepticism of workers who feel that the union movement is no longer relevant. In countries like Armenia, the Czech Republic, Poland and Lithuania, falling membership levels already challenge their claim to be the collective voice of health sector workers. This raises the spectre of unions being trapped in a downwards spiral, ruled out of negotiations on the grounds that their constituency is too small and becoming ever less relevant to their members because they are not full partners for social dialogue.

A modicum of hope is offered by the fact that however discredited unions may seem in some countries they are clearly sorely needed across the whole region. Workers may have expressed cynicism about their ability to deliver change but they were no less sceptical about the motives of government and employers (except perhaps in the Czech Republic). Indeed, they believed in significant numbers that management attitudes had hardened over recent years (fig. 27) and that plans already formulated by government would worsen their situation (fig. 28). The evidence of workers' disquiet suggests that unions do still have a constituency and a role to play. It confirms that trade unions should persist in seeking effective negotiating rights to address working conditions, job security and remuneration and in insisting that they are the most suitable and legitimate means of representing workers in social dialogue.

---

[96] Although the single largest response to the inquiry about changes in union strength was "do not know", 47.7 per cent of Ukrainian respondents, 39.4 per cent of Romanians, and 28.1 per cent of Lithuanians strongly agreed or agreed that their union had become less powerful in the last five years. The figure was only 12.6 per cent in the Czech Republic.

Corrosive reform: Failing health systems in Eastern Europe

Figure 27. Percentage of respondents who felt that management had become less concerned with the needs of workers over the previous five years

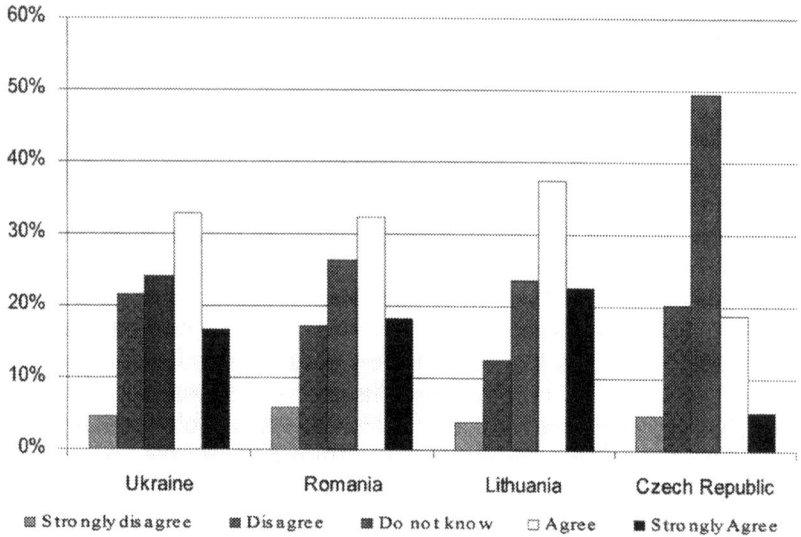

Source: (ILO, 2001).

Figure 28. Percentage of respondents who expected that existing government plans would make their job worse

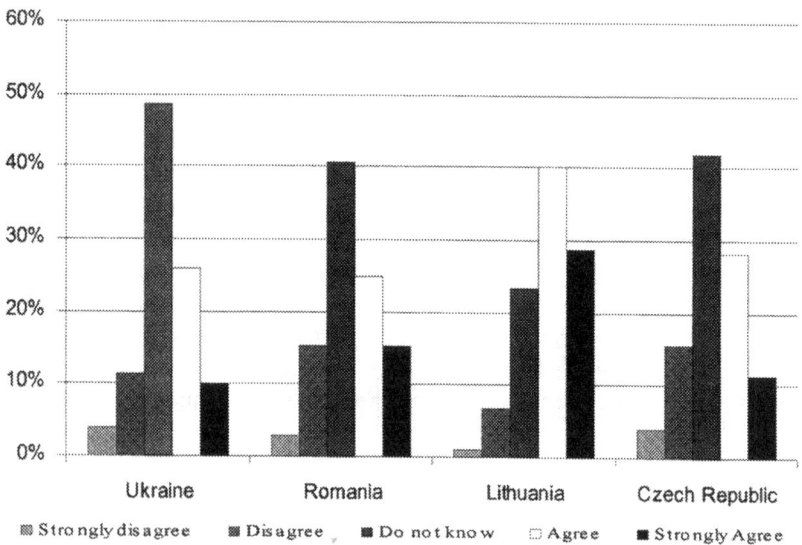

Source: (ILO, 2001).

Union functions: change, continuity and traditions under fire

What unions do now in seeking to address work, employment, job and income security is in many respects to continue those functions, which have always been at the conventional or traditional heart of trade unionism. It would be wrong however, to assume that the focus on the cornerstones of collective bargaining, wages and benefits implies straightforward continuity with the past. The extent of the change across CEE and CIS has forced a reworking of many of these roles so that current functions often have only a nominal relationship with those of the past. Bargaining for example, which was highly formulaic in the centrally planned economies has been transformed into all too real negotiations, with unions having to defend their right to be recognized as partners for social dialogue. Trade unions have had to adapt to these new demands and many have had to review which functions they can carry out. In countries like Armenia, Kyrgyzstan, or the Republic of Moldova they attempt to cover all areas while in Belarus and Lithuania unions are only in a position to discuss wages. In Slovakia and Russia, unions have managed to formalize their position in monitoring compliance with regulations on remuneration and conditions while in Belarus, Latvia and Ukraine they are directly involved in disbursing benefits. There are varying degrees of success in fulfilling these different functions across the region.

Unions do not appear to be enormously or uniformly successful in securing better pay (see income security). Although concessions and pay rises have been achieved in the public sector particularly in Moldova, Romania and Ukraine, pay in these cases is still startlingly low. This is no doubt mostly due to the resource constraints facing health care systems in CEE and CIS. It may also reflect the complexity of collective bargaining at national, provincial and hospital levels [97]. These multi-layered negotiations are a consequence of decentralization (see below) but have inevitably led to conflicting agreements and confusion that make it ever more difficult for unions to protect their members.

Traditionally unions were also active in guaranteeing working conditions and participated in joint health and safety committees. The decade after transition however, saw many of the provisions for management consultation fall into disuse. By 2000 it was commonplace for unions to be excluded from discussions of workplace safety or from playing a part in inspections (see work

---

[97] The ILO/PSI survey shows that the bulk of countries (Armenia, Belarus, Bulgaria, Georgia, Kyrgyzstan, Lithuania, the Republic of Moldova, Poland, and the Russian Federation) expected negotiations to take place at all three levels. In Latvia negotiations took place at the national and hospital levels and in the Czech Republic at the hospital level only. Bargaining is more centralized in Croatia and Slovakia and is at a national level only, although the Croatian governments unilateral decision to impose pay cuts in 1999 demonstrated the relative powerlessness of unions in such negotiations.

security). Negotiation of demarcation issues, the establishment of norms and the protection of skills and qualifications are other areas that would have fallen to unions in the past. There is little evidence to show that unions still play an active role in this respect and increasingly it is associations who are involved in determining where job boundaries lie through accreditation and licensing (see below). A somewhat similar process has taken place with regard to training, which is increasingly linked to professional bodies. Nonetheless, unions have a role albeit a diminished one and in Bulgaria, Latvia and Slovakia they all participate in training development (see skill reproduction security).

Another longstanding role of trade unions (and one which is now set in a startlingly different environment) has been to consult with national partners, most specifically Ministries of Health. It is unclear how influential such consultations would have been before transition but it is hard to believe that unions have more say now than they did then. Nonetheless, meetings have continued and seem to concentrate on core themes like wages, hours and training, although there are also reports of wider discussions around legislation and privatization. There are, however, vast differences across the region in how often discussions take place and how useful they are felt to be. In Poland for example, there are consultations every month, while in the Republic of Moldova meetings are only as and when needed. In Moldova they are considered to be constructive approximately 60 per cent of the time whereas in Lithuania consultations are considered useful only 6 per cent of the time. In the Russian Federation, the Ministry of Health seem to regard the dialogue as helpful while union members perceive no benefits as a result (see above).

Finally, the organization and coordination of industrial action might be included in a list of "traditional" union functions. This was not the case however, in CEE and CIS before transition, although the right to strike did exist. Nor is it generally the case in health sectors. On the whole health workers across the region are entitled to strike and only Bulgaria reported an outright ban [98], but despite difficult and worsening conditions it is still relatively uncommon, although not unheard of for staff to withdraw their labour [99]. PSI do report a considerable increase in strike action (by unions that have no tradition of leading strikes) but in these instances the withdrawal of labour has mostly been for short periods only. There may be several reasons for this reluctance to take (prolonged) strike action, but one is surely unwillingness on the part of staff to disrupt the care their patients receive. The fact that staff have a complex

---

[98] There were constraints on strike action for certain doctors in Poland and the Republic of Moldova, for doctors and nurses in Armenia and Slovakia and for nurses in the Russian Federation. Lithuania is introducing widespread restrictions, although the extent of these is still unclear (ILO, 2001).

[99] Workers in Georgia, the Republic of Moldova and Poland have all resorted to strike action albeit on a limited scale (Afford, 2001 and ILO, Domagala et al., 2000).

attachment to their work should not however be seen as indicating contentment. Unions have often been involved in organizing demonstrations to protest worsening conditions and low pay.

In all these instances the formal functions of trade unions are consistent with their roles before transition and with a "normal" range of union activities. There has been no radical overhaul in what workers' representatives aspire to do on behalf of staff. There has however, been a huge change in the world in which they operate. Not only are relations with governments and employers transformed by the shift to market economies but health systems restructuring has often made it difficult for national unions to operate effectively. What is more, unions must take on new tasks if they are to respond to the reforms around them. Commenting on draft laws or the implications of health insurance schemes, or representing staff in the face of restructuring initiatives or privatization go well beyond what unions "used to do". Union staff have little training or experience in these areas and there are not normally funds to employ specialists or lawyers. This makes it particularly difficult for them to expand their functions, to deliver expert leadership or to ensure the kind of security that staff need.

New unions, new associations: enhancing and undermining voice representation

As the traditional unions of CEE and CIS struggle with the challenges to their legitimacy posed by new health system structures, changing relations with government and falling membership, so they are confronted with new organizations seeking to represent workers. Although there are still countries like Belarus and the Republic of Moldova that have only one trade union covering the entire health sector workforce, there are more and more cases of new unions being founded to represent specific occupations or simply in order to break away from existing bodies. This type of proliferation has already occurred in Croatia, Lithuania and Poland (table 12).

The growth of new professional associations has been even more noticeable than the growth of new unions. They are identified by a variety of terms (associations, societies, chambers) but all seek to represent and protect the interests of a single occupational group or a coalition of linked groups within health. The majority focus on physicians or specialist sub-groups of physicians. Nonetheless there were associations for a full range of occupational groups including pharmacists and paramedics (table 13), although these are less powerful on the whole.

Corrosive reform: Failing health systems in Eastern Europe

Table 12.   New trade unions, Lithuania and Poland, 2001

Lithuania	Union of Doctors-Managers of Lithuania
	Trade Union of Health Workers of Lithuania
	Trade Union of Doctors-Administrators of Health Sector of Lithuania
	Union of Young Doctors of Lithuania
	Trade Union of Medical Workers of Lithuania
	Union of Nurses of Lithuania
	Lithuanian Trade Union of Specialist in Taking Care of the Sick
	Association under the Health Department of Lithuania
Poland	National Trade Union of Solidarnosc
	National Trade Union of Physicians
	National Trade Union of Anaesthesia workers
	National Trade Union of Nurses and Midwives
	National Trade Union of Technicians
	National Trade Union of Radiology workers
	National Trade Union of Dentistry workers

Source: (Afford, 2001 and ILO, 2001 survey responses).

Table 13.   New forms of voice representation, Slovakia, 2001

Trade unions	Slovak Trade Union of Health
	Medical Trade Union Associations
Professional bodies	Slovak Medical Chamber
	Slovak Chamber of Dentists
	Slovak Pharmaceutical Chamber
	Slovak Chamber of Paramedical Personnel (covering nurses, laboratory technicians and other paramedical staff)
	Slovak Chamber of University Graduated Health Workers
Associations	Association of Hospitals of Slovakia
	Association of Independent Polyclinics
	Association of Middle Health Schools
	Association of State Health Institutes
	Association of Private Doctors

Source: (Afford, 2001 and ILO, 2001 survey responses).

Table 14.   Membership of associations and trade unions, selected countries, 2001

Country	Level of membership (in percentage)	
	Associations	Trade unions
Latvia	60.0	50.2
Lithuania	85.0	20.0
Republic of Moldova	79.0	89.2
Poland	40–45	20.0
The Russian Federation	80.3	81.2
Slovakia	80.0	75.2

Source: Afford, 2001 and ILO, 2001 survey responses.

The growth of new unions and associations offers representation security to some, very particular groups. While all legitimate representative voices ought to be heard, the tendency of the more powerful and better-paid groups to peel off from mainstream unions must undermine the representation security of the health workforce as a whole. At the very least fragmentation will distract from the core messages and at worst different sectional groups will be pitted against each other with the strongest professions (the doctors) winning out at the expense of the weaker majority [100].

The impact of health system reforms on voice representation

It has been said many times, and is no less true for that, that if reforms in the health sector are to be successful they must involve and motivate those people who will implement them [101]. Social dialogue in the hospital sector is particularly important because of the labour intensive nature of services and the challenges of EU enlargement [102]. Yet despite the fact that the case for the inclusion of workers' representatives in reforms has been made (and accepted) over and over again there has been an extraordinary lack of genuine consultation in CEE and CIS. Reforms to the structure, organization and management of health services have been undertaken without proper reference to unions as barometers of workers' opinions, and in particular without reference to the implications they will have for the long-term security of voice representation in the health sector.

Decentralization is a case in point. It is one of the most widespread reforms of the last decade and has included variously, a shift of funding and management responsibilities from central to local government, the introduction of insurance funds and the empowerment of hospitals, and more particularly hospital directors [103]. While it may have helped health care management to be closer to the needs of the patient it has left unions (and associations) struggling to cope with fragmented employment and a myriad of governmental levels, institutions and small practices all employing staff directly. While government is still the largest single employer, the impact of "more independently acting employers

---

[100] Already, there are examples of doctors' associations and physicians' chambers advocating privatization policies that are to their own advantage but which jeopardize the security of most workers and threaten to restrict access to health care.

[101] Ottawa Charter for Health Promotion 1986, WHO World Health Report 2000, World Bank cited in Afford (2001) amongst others.

[102] Declaration from the Second Conference on the Social Dialogue in the Hospital Sector in Europe — Brussels 4 and 5 February 2002, as it appears in ILO (2000a).

[103] Of the 15 countries in the ILO/PSI survey only Belarus and Ukraine failed to identify decentralization as a reform of major importance for the country.

striving at efficiency under local conditions" is immense (ILO, 2002a, p. 51). It has led to disruption in a number of areas, not least because "the cooperation and coordination with similar public or semi-public employers still have to be created in many countries" (ILO, 2002a). There are no adequate structures in place to ensure that workers in all institutions and at all levels are guaranteed a voice.

Collective bargaining has already suffered (see above). It is not however, a simple case of uncertainty as unions try to establish the relative authority of different levels of local, regional and national management. It is also about levels of competence. Unions are often confronted with inability on the part of decentralized bodies to meet their responsibilities. This sometimes reflects a lack of skills and training at the regional, or establishment level since staff in new organizations are not all equipped to take on the roles of director, head of finance or human resources manager [104]. It is more often the result of indebtedness. Where resources are insufficient to sustain the immediate decentralization of the health care system, then union negotiations on pay and conditions become meaningless. A hospital owed money by insurance companies and on the verge of bankruptcy will not increase remuneration [105].

Decentralization has also led to a marked decline in equity as pay disparities have opened up between regions with different levels of resources at their disposal. There is also evidence of inequities emerging between staff in different sectors and from different occupational groups (Afford, 2001). There are even examples of staff carrying out similar jobs in the same hospital being employed on different contract types and receiving different pay. All of these demonstrate how far the achievements of the union movement have been rolled back, particularly in countries that have devolved the right to set pay and benefit levels to individual hospital directors. Small units, like single-handed general practices or small group dental practices which employ support and auxiliary staff directly present a similar threat to collective voice representation. This is not to suggest that either hospital directors or general practitioners will undermine income or representation security maliciously. It is more that as employers allocating limited resources they are likely to prioritize patient care, or their own income, at the expense of staff pay. Unions will inevitably find it extremely difficult to intervene on behalf of staff in this kind of setting.

Unions are also likely to find it difficult to represent and protect staff as performance related pay and incentives are introduced. It is acknowledged that "performance appraisal as a tool of performance management has to be related to incentives but it also has to be secure against potential abuse by those who use this instrument" (ILO, 2002a, p. 15). Many unions are poorly placed to negotiate

---

[104] The role of unions in identifying skills gaps and in ensuring staff have access to adequate training has already been discussed in Sections 5 and 6 Job and Skill Reproduction Security.

[105] This precise scenario is cited by the Lithuania respondent to the ILO/PSI survey.

the parameters of the system or police it and associations are unlikely to be even-handed in addressing the implications of any bonus schemes.

The introduction of social insurance has already been referred to. It is a form of decentralization that involves vesting governmental responsibilities as third party payer in quasi-autonomous bodies and is common in CEE and in parts of the former Soviet Union. It is implicated in problems of indebtedness but has additional implications for traditional collective arrangements. Specifically, insurance mechanisms invite experimentation with pay formulae, especially payments made to physicians. It is not necessarily the case that these will undercut previous arrangements, it is likely though that in many cases they will result in the exclusion of trade unions from the negotiating process. There is already evidence that professional associations are the preferred partners of insurance companies in consultations on remuneration (see above) and this bodes ill for all other occupational groups who are not represented and for unions' role in future discussions of payment structures [106].

Privatization is another of the reforms, which has decentralized authority and simultaneously challenged voice representation. There are few data from the private sector but it seems that attitudes to unions are more negative than in the public sector. Unionization rates may also be lower, if only because so much of the private sector is made up of small establishments like dentists' practices, pharmacies and diagnostic clinics, while the unions of CEE and CIS have always been geared up to work in the public sector with its standard employment contracts and large institutions. There must be real concern as to how unions will begin to adapt their structures and processes to address the representation needs of staff in small and perhaps isolated private units, and how if at all, they will cope with the self-employed.

Privatization also raises the spectre of sub-contracting. Evidence from Western Europe suggests that "relatively small operational units of health services at local government levels, (that have) a lack of critical mass in delivering or in purchasing services ... (have) led to contracting out certain services, such as cleaning, catering and information technology" (ILO, 2002a, p. 51). There is little evidence to date on contracting out in CEE or CIS but Western experience suggests it represents a significant blow to voice representation with the firms that take on contracts for hotel services typically resisting unionization and collective bargaining [107].

---

[106] The fact that they do not have experience in this kind of negotiation does not help their position but the key to their exclusion will surely be the narrow sectional interest of the physicians' associations and the lack of interest on the part of third-party payers in negotiating with a wide spectrum of health sector staff.

[107] There is also compelling evidence that contracting out leads to worsening of pay and conditions and a decline in trust between employers and employees (Hunter, 1998).

It is perhaps worth mentioning here that despite all the reforms taking place, the withdrawal of central government from many areas of employment and the emergence of a range of organizational forms there are still very few distinct, clearly identifiable and formally constituted bodies representing the new employers. The autonomous management of hospitals and clinics are of course "real" but they are not yet well enough established to have agreed on a means of articulating a shared voice. This makes it all the harder for trade unions to identify who to negotiate with and on what basis. Where they can no longer dialogue with government there is as yet no obvious alternative.

Unions, social dialogue and the scope for a constructive future

The role of trade unions has been under attack from all directions. Health systems have experienced economic crises of unprecedented depths. Resource constraints combined with the sheer pace of the changes taking place, have made it more and more difficult for unions to fulfil their traditional or their new functions. Health system reforms have fragmented the workforce and created new employers confusing the relationships between them and upsetting established bargaining mechanisms. International organizations and donors have also played a part in undermining the collective voice, promoting models of reform that ignore representation security and actively discourage the proper incorporation of trade unions into social dialogue (Standing, 1997, p. 1349).

There is nonetheless, a positive and valuable role for workers' representatives. Just as professional associations are taking on statutory responsibilities in determining professional standards so trade unions should be formally incorporated into the policy-making process with regard to all aspects of employment. The development of tripartite boards, in place of the old command-transmission mechanisms, could furnish unions with just such a role, although the boards will have little positive impact if their agendas and the decisions taken are not relevant and acceptable to all parties (Standing, 1996, p. 249). The approach to social dialogue needs to be managed with care therefore and planned and carried out with the genuine involvement of all appropriate parties (national, regional or local) at all appropriate stages (ILO, 2002b). Unions already have the capacity to understand and represent issues in a local setting or at a national level and are ideally placed to tailor their involvement to any stage of the negotiations. It will be important that governments too commit inputs at a relevant level and are willing to cut across sector boundaries to involve "ministries in charge of finance, planning, economic development and education" when needed (ILO, 2002a, p. 44). Similarly, where decentralization has devolved responsibilities to agencies like insurance funds, or indeed fund holding GPs, they will need to be included while "dialogue with user organizations and other stakeholders should also be encouraged where it is appropriate" (ILO, 2002b).

Hungary established just such a consultative mechanism in 1992 (the now defunct Interest Reconciliation Council for Budgetary Institutions). It acted as a negotiating forum for public services, including health and demonstrated that unions had an important part to play, alongside central and local government, in concluding agreements on issues like job classification and salary scales, and in discussing draft legislation [108]. The structures for conducting social dialogue may vary, but the Joint Meeting on Social Dialogue in the Health Services (Geneva 2002) concluded that when appropriately managed it is key in bringing "governments, employers and workers' organizations and other policy leaders to draw upon their knowledge and experience" to address structural change, quality and performance. This position is well supported by evidence from Zambia, which suggests that certain conditions must always be met if social dialogue is to guarantee a satisfactory voice for health sector employees. There needs to be a genuine commitment on the part of all partners (a national will to engage), clear agendas that meet national priorities, and the appropriate involvement of all the relevant and interrelated levels (Fashoyin, 2002, pp. 70–75). There must also be "strong, independent and responsible social partners" able and willing to participate (Fashoyin, 2002). The scope for trade union participation is clear. The success of their contribution will depend on whether or not they can stand up to the threats they face and maintain their claim to be strong, independent and valid social partners.

Conclusions and policy recommendations

Two things are eminently clear. First, trade unions have lost ground over the last decade. Second, they are needed more than ever. The conditions health sector workers face can only be addressed by a collective voice but in many respects unions are caught in a cleft stick. They need to maintain high membership levels if they are to be able to claim legitimately that they represent health service workers and in order to be recognized as the leading partners for social dialogue. However, health sector staff are discouraged from continuing in membership because unions have been overlooked by government and decentralized layers of health services management and have played little part in formulating health sector reforms. Workers are increasingly faced with the proposition of ever increasing amounts of their pay (bonuses and incentives schemes) being determined exclusively by management and insurance companies and without reference to their union representatives.

It has also been difficult for unions to demonstrate their effectiveness because of the scale of the upheaval that has affected health systems. Levels of pay, the investment in infrastructure that determines working conditions, the availability of training, even changing contract types have all been beyond the locus of control of Ministries of Health, let alone health unions. Furthermore

---

[108] For full account, see ILO (2002a, p. 41).

Corrosive reform: Failing health systems in Eastern Europe

Ministries have often withdrawn from their role as employer before any effective "replacement" has emerged. Employers are poorly defined and poorly organized and unions have had few effective counterparts. They cannot therefore, be deemed to have failed because they could not deliver the impossible.

The position has not been helped by the legacy of distrust that some unions inherited from the pre-transition period, when they could be viewed as too close to central government and the communist party. Nor has the growth of professional associations reinforced a collective voice rather they have undermined it. It is of course legitimate for professions to organize independently and secure their own representation, and many members of associations continue to belong to unions. Nonetheless, the breach in the solidarity between professionals and unskilled staff that existed in the era of single, general unions is to be regretted.

The negativity of some international agencies and donors has helped to exclude unions from playing a part in developing plans for reform, and what is more has ensured that they were seen to be excluded. This will jeopardize the reforms themselves, which will be formulated without the benefit of union participation and "buy-in", and without drawing on the wealth of experience and understanding that health care system workers could contribute. It will also further undermine the credibility of unions. Certain donors may not like unions but if they succeed in undermining their viability they risk utterly destroying voice representation and the overall sustainability of the reforms. This would not only have adverse implications for a whole range of elements of socio-economic security (job, work, income etc.) but would also be profoundly negative, in and of itself, unless of course the international community would regard it as acceptable that the health workforce of Eastern Europe were denied a collective voice.

Public Services International has suggested trade unions "as workers' representatives must demand to be treated as genuine social partners in all major social-economic planning and decision making. Full social dialogue. Nothing less. If these principles are respected by the government, then trade unions can consider any proposition because they will be able to negotiate in an atmosphere of genuine social partnership" [109].

This captures the need to place unions at the heart of efforts to shape health systems so that they provide the best possible care for patients and look after the well-being of their staff. Although there can be no guarantees that unions will be allowed this role, the following recommendations outline some possible steps towards achieving the vision touched on by PSI.

International agencies and bilateral assistance programmes should:

---

[109] PSI Policy Statement on Social Dialogue, quoted in ILO (2002a).

- review their thinking on the importance of social dialogue;

- make a formal commitment to fostering and working within tripartite structures that wholeheartedly include trade unions;

- advocate for governments to make a corresponding commitment;

- encourage national unions to review the situation analyses and country reports that provide the basis for developing aid and loan agreements;

- invite national unions to comment on aid and loan agreements before signature (incorporating their feedback into revised proposals);

- support research into levels of unionization and de-unionization in the private sector, and in parallel health systems and into social dialogue;

- sponsor a review of the impact of trade union support on the implementation of policy recommendations; and

- provide the resources for and facilitate the training of mangers and union representatives in social dialogue.

Governments should:

- establish tripartite structures that include trade unions and all other relevant social partners, and ensure the involvement of all levels and branches of government and health service management;

- lobby extensively to build genuine acceptance of the social dialogue approach;

- develop specific and appropriate priorities for the tripartite structures to address and monitor progress against agreed agendas;

- pass legislation enshrining the right to union membership and for unions to be recognized by employers, with special reference to the private sector, to parallel health services and to small establishments like general or dental practices;

- work with unions and professional associations to identify mechanisms which will ensure full representation for an increasingly disaggregated workforce;

- reassert the role of collective bargaining, confirming the statutory role of unions in national and sub-national negotiations and as the partner of government;

- clarify the jurisdictions of different levels of management, particularly in terms of collective bargaining;

- balance the role of professional associations (in standard setting, training and negotiations on remuneration and bonuses) with proper consultation with unions and mandate insurance bodies to do likewise; and

- maintain and strengthen existing bipartite structures at enterprise level to ensure full consultation on the details of specific issues relating to work, job, employment and skill reproduction security.

Trade unions should:

- ensure that they reach out to all staff and in all employment settings, including in small decentralized units, private and single-handed practices and in the parallel health services;

- review internal structures and processes and adapt them as necessary to facilitate the involvement of staff employed in the private sector and in small employment units;

- identify and mobilize staff whose careers are under threat from modernization either of institutional or career structures, lobbying to ensure they are re-trained and otherwise properly supported in making a transition to a new employment setting;

- seek to motivate and encourage health service workers to join and take an active part in trade union activities, making particular efforts to adapt internal processes and structures so that they empower women and to incorporate their concerns and priorities into bargaining strategies;

- identify and link up with Western European unions who have effectively tackled falling membership to identify strategies that will ensure their relevance to workers and attract new and active members;

- liase with international organizations, academia and non-governmental organizations (particularly where they are committed to securing access to health care services for populations) to secure the skilled and expert inputs needed to respond to proposed reforms and suggested structural changes;

- demand clarity about the level at which collective bargaining will be carried out and insist on binding agreements;

- establish links with health insurance bodies and other third party payers insisting on equal rights to associations in all negotiations and convincing associations to hold joint negotiations;

- champion social dialogue across the health sector; and

- comment actively on loans and demand a role in the negotiation of aid and loan packages.

INCOME SECURITY [110]

9

Health service staff are poorly paid in much of Europe and health workers in the CEE and CIS are no exception. They express an overwhelming dissatisfaction with salary levels (fig. 29) and although dissatisfaction on the part of staff does not prove that pay levels are inadequate, the evidence of genuine income insecurity and hardship is utterly compelling. Low pay in the sector is a long-standing feature and reflects the value attached to health service work before transition [111] as well as the collapse in the value of public expenditures over the past decade. It is also testament to the fact that policy-makers and international financial institutions still will not prioritize health care systems. There is little evidence that the position is improving markedly or equitably, even though many of the region's economies have been growing over recent years [112]. (Although doctors in one or two countries like the Czech Republic or Poland have secured significant increases, most occupations have not).

This section examines health sector pay and the paucity of formal income levels, which may encourage staff to seek work in Western Europe. It touches on the problems of payment in arrears, and the inadequacy of benefits and pensions. It reflects on the fact that the monetarization of in-kind benefits has made staff ever more vulnerable to under-investment in the health sector and reviews further evidence of insecurity, provided by data on overtime worked and the numbers of staff holding second jobs. It also discusses the importance of informal gratitude or under-the-table payments. It concludes that the reforms that health systems have undergone have exacerbated rather than resolved problems of income security not least because they have focused on ways of manipulating performance, redefining workers' roles and cutting costs rather than looking at the people who work in health. It suggests that the focus on controlling outputs and on the payment of doctors as a key lever for achieving this control has

---

[110] The IFP/SES defines Income Security as protection of income through minimum wage, wage indexation, comprehensive social security, progressive taxation, etc.

[111] Health sector pay was traditionally low because working in health was considered "unproductive" and was therefore less well remunerated than "productive" work such as manufacturing. The fact that the majority of the workforce was (and still is) female both reflects this and compounds the situation.

[112] The fact that there are so many women in the health workforce has not helped prompt a readjustment.

disadvantaged the majority of health sector staff, and ultimately the users of health care services.

Figure 29. Percentage of staff that agreed they were happy with their current pay

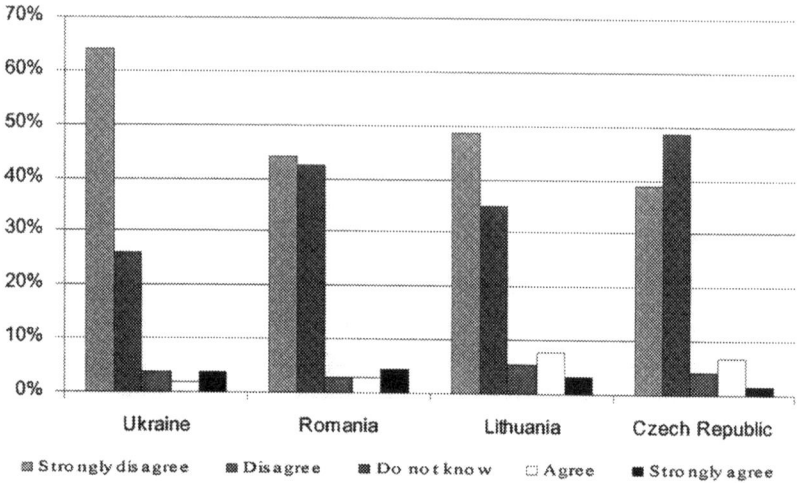

Source: (ILO, 2001).

Low pay — less pay: palpable insecurity

Low wages are endemic to health sectors across the region and feature particularly in those countries that spend the lowest percentage of their GDP on health [113]. It is commonplace for health workers' pay to be held at or below the minimum wage (table 15), and again this practice is most widespread in the former Soviet Union and Central Asia. The use of the minimum wage is significant because although it was intended to be (and once was) a source of basic income security, it has been turned into a de-facto "mechanism of destitution", by policy-makers who are conscious both of the number of public sector staff on minimum pay and of the way benefit levels are tied to it [114]. In order to restrict public expenditures they have allowed the minimum wage to fall drastically behind national average incomes, effectively making it a source of poverty. This has transformed the notion of what it is to be poor in CEE and CIS. It was something that affected only vulnerable groups or those who did not

---

[113] It is difficult to measure the percentage of GDP spent on health with any accuracy as informal payments make up a significant part of expenditure. Estimates by WHO, the UNDP and the World Bank suggest that the countries of the central Asia and the Caucasus, as well as Belarus, the Republic of Moldova, Romania, the Russian Federation and Ukraine are the most catastrophically affected with expenditure falling to levels where it genuinely interferes with the ability of the health system to perform. See Afford (2001) and WHO (2001b) for more details.

[114] For details of the minimum wage see Standing (1997, p. 1348).

work but as Standing points out now, "unlike the past, a high proportion of the poor are working poor" [115].

Table 15. Percentage of workforce paid at or below the minimum wage, selected countries

	Percentage of workforce paid at or below the minimum wage
Armenia	30 per cent
Bulgaria	25 per cent a rise from 1996 when only 20 per cent were affected
Georgia	90 per cent of staff in the public sector 50 per cent of staff in the private sector
Latvia	2.3 per cent of staff in the public sector 13.9 per cent of staff in the private sector
Poland	70 per cent

Source: (Afford, 2001).

The ILO/PSI survey confirms that the income of Russian and Moldovan health sector staff (in all occupations) has fallen relative to the national average wage and that in Armenia and Belarus falls have affected all medical professions (Afford, 2001). Stepantchikova confirms this picture (table 16). However, even in countries where there is no explicit link between health services pay and the minimum wage the sector routinely sets wage levels below the national average. In Lithuania for example, health workers' average salaries were only 83 per cent of the national average, while in Bulgaria the relative pay of all groups except doctors has fallen against the national average (ILO, 2001). This reflects not only the poor (low paid) starting point of the health sector but also it's weak bargaining power compared to other sectors that can demonstrate more clearly their contribution to economic growth [116]. It may also be that the traditional reluctance of health system staff to take prolonged and disruptive industrial action allows their claim to a greater share of public resources to be more easily overlooked. Certainly the fact that the health sector caters to many of the most vulnerable (and least influential) groups in society and that in so much of CEE and CIS the more affluent can secure preferential treatment through formal or informal out-of-pocket payments does little to strengthen the position of health sector staff in negotiating better pay.

[115] Standing (1997, p. 1345) who cites evidence that "In both Poland and Russia a majority of the poor have been nominally in employment" (*The World Bank (1996)*, p. 15, 115).

[116] Although health is an important contributor to development, most national policy-makers view it as a drain on resources rather than an engine for growth (WHO, 2002a).

Table 16.   Average monthly salary in health care as a percentage of the average monthly salary in all sectors, 1961–2000

Year	1961	1970	1980	1990	1992	1999*	2000*
	72	75	75	68	64	51	46

* Parliamentary Hearings "Socio-Economic Status of Health Care Workers", April 12–13, 2000, in Stepantchikova *et al.* (2001).

Source: Government Report on Health Care, 1992, page 110.

Evidence on health sector pay relative to average pay highlights the problem of falling income over time and certainly nominal increases in income have not always translated into rising purchasing power. Recent wage increases in Georgia, Kyrgyzstan and Moldova for example, have done little to offset the strains of purchasing food, housing, heating and other utilities in increasingly deregulated markets, and in all three countries the rises are reported not to have lifted the majority of health workers above subsistence level income. Large numbers of health workers, including many in CEE, have suffered a fall in real wages over the past decade as inflation has devalued their pay and as market economies have consolidated, eating into those areas of service provision where workers might previously have received de facto subsidy from the public purse.

A review of cash remuneration alone does not capture the full impact of inflation on income security. "Crèches, holiday homes, clinics, sports facilities, training institutes, schools, rented housing, and enterprise shops providing subsidized consumer goods" were all part of the effort made in centrally planned economies to replace monetary rewards with non-cash benefits {see employment security} (Standing, 1997, p. 1346). There has been rapid and widespread erosion of these in-kind benefits. Some have been lost altogether and those still in place are mostly less comprehensive and of lower quality, reducing the value of the remuneration staff receive markedly. This is not just a blow to overall income but has also meant an increased reliance on cash earnings for staff at precisely the time when the real value of cash payments has been falling and the cost of buying services in the market place has escalated (Standing, 1997, pp. 1343–1346).

Workers' perceptions are that they experience an absolute lack of security and relative disadvantage. An appallingly high number of staff in the four-country survey (between 60 and 80 per cent) worried that they could not live on their wages (fig. 30), while the vast majority in Lithuania, Romania and Ukraine believed that they earned less than five years before (fig. 31). The extent of the fear that workers live with is hard to comprehend and is absolutely inimical to income security [117]. It must encourage them to consider migrating to wealthier countries within the region or to Western Europe in search of better-paid work.

---

[117] Even in the few cases where doctors have secured advantageous terms (and in the Czech Republic they earn twice the national average salary) they still report concerns and insecurity.

Not all occupational groups however, experience income insecurity equally. Reductions in pay compared to national average wages have been uneven across occupational boundaries. Typically physicians have fared better than their co-workers and this is in no small part due to the emphasis of policy-makers on doctors and their performance, coupled with the success of their newly established professional associations. A widening pay gap has certainly been a feature in Belarus, Bulgaria, Croatia and the Czech Republic. That differentials should have increased over the past ten years was perhaps to be expected. The extent to which they have grown however, may well breed resentment and demoralization in the sector. What is also striking is how inequities have widened not just on the basis of occupation but also as a result of the ability of employers to pay. In the Russian Federation some parallel health care systems (specifically that of the Ministry of Defence) are able to afford significantly more than the United Tariff Scale for mainstream services while 'geographic' allowances paid in more affluent areas have introduced significant gaps between pay in different parts of the country [118].

Figure 30. **Percentage of staff who agreed that the ability to live on their wages was one of their greatest worries**

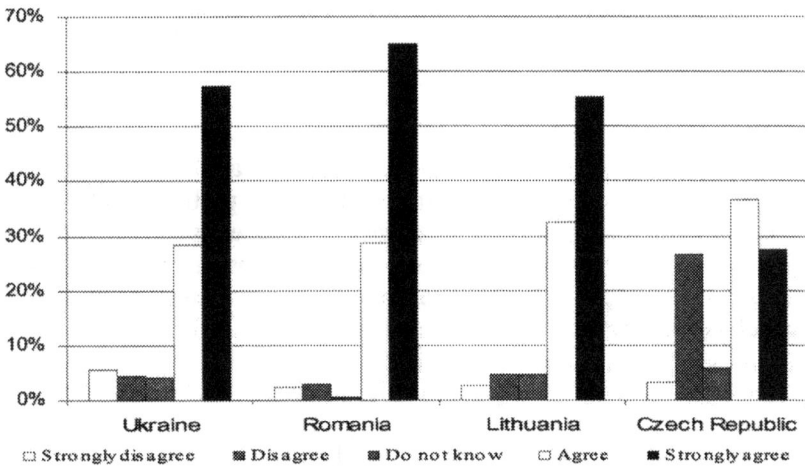

Source: (ILO, 2001)

---

[118] For details see Stepantchikova *et al.* (2001).

Figure 31. Percentage of staff that felt that after taking inflation into account they were paid less than five years before

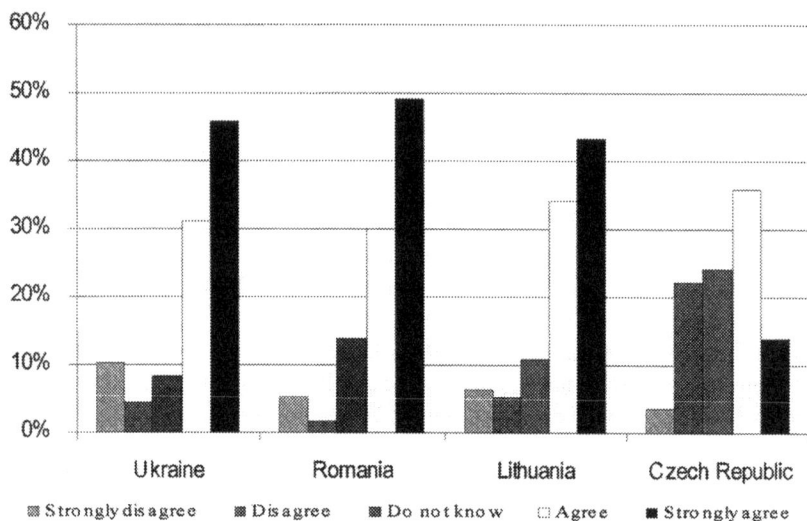

Source: (ILO, 2001).

Paid late — if paid at all

The paucity of income for many (in cash and in-kind) is made all but insufferable for some by wage arrears. This is a problem that was powerfully associated with the economic collapse of the early 1990s and which was particularly prevalent in the former Soviet Union. It persists today and still seems to be largely if not exclusively, a phenomenon of former Soviet Republics, despite the fact that many have ratified ILO Convention 101, which stipulates that wages should be paid on time. The ILO/PSI survey found that in the months leading up to the survey 100 per cent of Armenian workers received at least some of their wages late, whilst in Moldova and Georgia three quarters and one half of workers respectively had part of their wage payment delayed. The situation is also reported to be particularly severe in rural areas of the Ukraine while in the Russian Federation employers had an outstanding wage bill of 238.1 million Roubles as of February 2001 [119]. The four-country survey confirms that the problem continues to affect the region and that over a third of workers in Lithuania and Ukraine experienced delays in receiving their full pay (fig. 32).

---

[119] A significant improvement on the 4.5 billion roubles owed in 1999. See Stepantchikova *et al.* (2001).

Figure 32. Percentage of staff that had experience of not receiving their full pay on time

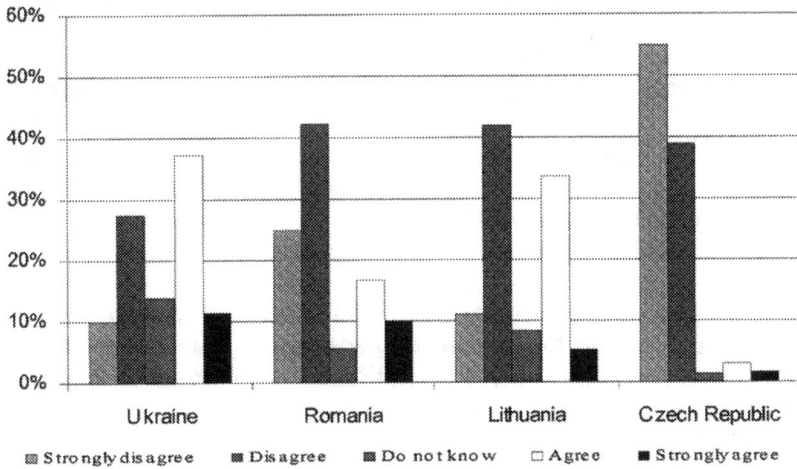

Legend: ▨ Strongly disagree ▨ Disagree ▦ Do not know ▢ Agree ■ Strongly agree

Source: (ILO, 2001).

Delaying payments to staff is not the same as putting them on administrative leave [120] (although there is a degree of overlap) but both result, at least in part, from a "tightening (of) social budgets (that) has resulted in widespread and serious "wage arrears" in the public health care system" and both hugely compromise an employee's choices (Standing, 1996, p. 246). Administrative leave has already been shown to trap workers in poverty and to undermine their entitlement to benefit or to disentitle them altogether [121]. Delays in payment have a similar effect. They force employees to live on below subsistence incomes and deny them access to benefits. They also make it extremely difficult to move on, since workers cannot be expected to walk away from employers that owe them money. The boundaries between these two forms of income insecurity are not always clear-cut, but the negative consequences for staff of either one could not be more obvious.

Not only do wages go unpaid but benefit and pension obligations are not always honoured. Most of the region lacks comprehensive social security and limits the availability of crucial welfare benefits and evidence from the ILO–PSI survey suggests that health workers are even worse of in practice than on paper. Although their entitlements are underwritten by nationally agreed regulations

[120] Administrative leave has already been fully discussed in Section 3 Labour Market Security.

[121] Employers can obstruct workers trying to secure severance pay and there are also barriers to benefit for those "making themselves voluntarily unemployed", which put workers under pressure to accept administrative leave. However, employees may also forego their right to severance pay because they can subsist on in-kind benefits and feel that these are more secure than unemployment benefits. It is unclear what will happen as the value of non-monetary benefits diminishes further.

(rather than local agreements), in reality neither government nor enterprise-derived benefits are always made available to them. Unemployment benefits have been pushed down in value, often under pressure from international agencies such as the World Bank, and have been reformed to restrict entitlement whilst maternity, disability and other benefits have failed to keep pace with rising costs {see employment security} (Standing, 1996, pp.236–237). The introduction of short-term employment contracts can only exacerbate the situation, undermining the rights of "temporary" staff to enterprise-based benefits and making it unlikely that the "casual" labour force will ever be able to secure entitlement to unemployment benefits.

Just as benefits (in many countries) cannot provide security for staff, so pensions are not able to guarantee an adequate income. It was commonplace for retired staff in CEE and CIS to continue in employment during the communist period and this is still the case; a testament to the ongoing problems of low-pay and low benefit levels (see work security). This is made worse in parts of the former Soviet Union by the long delays pensioners have experienced in receiving pension payments and by changes in entitlement in the Russian Federation that have reduced the pension rights of many staff (for details see Stepantchikova et al., 2001). There is some evidence in the ILO/PSI survey that countries are trying to address pension issues for the future but coverage is far from universal and provision seems unlikely to be adequate [122]. Given the emphasis in so many countries on cutting state spending, private and supplementary pension schemes will inevitably come under consideration. The implications of this policy shift for equity are worrying in the extreme. How staff who do not have even basic income security will be able to pay for adequate pension cover remains to be seen.

The insecurity of supplementary and informal payments

Large numbers of staff work overtime hours and many take on second jobs (see labour market and work security). Roughly a third of wages for doctors in Armenia, Belarus, Kyrgyzstan and the Russian Federation and a similar per cent of the pay of other occupations in Belarus and Kyrgyzstan are derived from second jobs [123] while Russian medical staff routinely occupy a series of part-time posts, or work privately after hours (for details see Stepantchikova et al., 2001). Staff seem to regard these additional commitments as normal or even essential parts of working life despite the impact they must have on their families. This provides compelling evidence that pay is too low to support workers or to

---

[122] It is as low as 20 per cent in Poland, ILO/PSI survey.

[123] ILO/PSI Survey.

provide them with adequate income security [124]. What is more, these patterns of work fuel a cycle of income insecurity. Overtime and extra jobs simply are not dependable sources of earnings but rather perpetuate the precarious element of remuneration in the health sector.

Informal payments for health care are similar in that they point to insecurity and help to create it. The nature of gratitude or under-the-table payments makes them difficult to quantify but they are clearly still common, in many parts of the region. WHO suggest that in Romania 30 per cent of health sector expenditure is informal, while the World Bank estimate that 78 per cent of spending is by individuals rather than from governmental sources and that only some of this is through formal co-payments. Reports from Armenia, Belarus, Kyrgyzstan, the Republic of Moldova and the Russian Federation, Bulgarian and Russian household surveys, and the reluctance of workers to be absent from work (see work security) all suggest an extensive reliance on direct payments in cash or kind from patients to staff, or from patients' relatives to staff [125, 126].

This is of real concern to health system planners who are charged with ensuring equity of access to services. It should be of equal concern to them that so many staff need to supplement their income and that so many staff are forced to depend on inherently unstable sources of pay. The effect of under-the-table payments on staff should not be underestimated and goes well beyond their unreliability. Staff are dependent on the means of the local population and so are faced with inequalities in pay between regions. Even more importantly under-the-table payments will tend to exacerbate pay differentials and inequalities between occupational groups. So staff with most patient contact and most influence over patient outcomes (doctors and some nurses) will be advantaged relative to "back room" staff such as administrators, and no doubt cleaners. This will further depress the income of the low paid relative to the wealthiest employees. Under-the-table payments are also likely to undermine wage negotiations since employers will inevitably be aware of the additional earnings and will take them into consideration when bargaining (offering less to offset the informal element of income). Furthermore while staff may benefit from under-the-table payments in the short-term, benefit and pension levels will not take them into account. This means that staff taking leave with benefits or retiring will be likely to experience a more significant drop in income than is officially the case, since their benefit or pension will be determined with reference to formal pay only.

---

[124] It also calls into question the assumptions about labour slack so common amongst international agencies.

[125] See Stepantchikova *et al.* (2001).

[126] For a fuller discussion of out-of-pocket and under-the-table payments see Afford (2001).

The problems that these payments hint at (low pay) and the problems that they cause (inequity and instability to name just two) are not of course easy to solve. While staff are inadequately paid and suffer regular wage arrears, there can be little incentive for them to give up an income stream which has long been a feature of the health sector and which may be culturally accepted. (Many patients appear comfortable with, or at least resigned to, the concept of giving the doctor a "present" to show appreciation and ensure quality of service.) Nonetheless, the range of disadvantages to staff (as well as patients) of relying of informal payments, not least the enormous income insecurity associated with them, must prompt health care systems to do better.

Reforming in income insecurity

Income insecurity stems in part, from the lack of resources in the health sector, exacerbated by the fact that in many CEE and CIS countries civil society still does not function as it should. This means low compliance in paying tax and insurance contributions and therefore a small pot of public monies from which to pay for all public sector expenditures. Notwithstanding the resource constraints much of the insecurity actually stems from a failure to prioritize and manage staff needs effectively. Reforms have been designed with reference to health systems literature but have not sought to address the consequences for staff of any of the proposed changes. This has led inevitably to unintended and negative outcomes from the employment perspective, which will without doubt undercut the intended benefits of the reforms.

Decentralization, as ever, provides ample illustration of how well meaning reforms can introduce insecurity for staff. Many of the countries of the region, encouraged by international agencies, prioritized decentralization as a means of enhancing efficiency and better responding to patient needs. The running of health services has therefore, been devolved to the regions, hospitals and clinics to varying degrees. This put much of the traditional national, collective bargaining process in jeopardy, inviting individual institutions and hospital directors to set wages and establish incentive schemes and allowing indebted institutions responsibilities for pay and pay negotiations. This was not of course an objective of the reform but does threaten national wage structures, (while increasing the need for a national system that can protect under-represented workers in small employment units). If national structures do break down, staff will come under pressure to "respond" to local conditions, which in poor regions could involve pay cuts that will increase inequities. Evidence of the negative impact of decentralization is already apparent in the Czech Republic where there are reports of migration between hospitals (albeit on a small scale) due to different wages and conditions (ILO, 2001) and in Poland where staff in the same hospital doing similar jobs may now be employed by different levels of government [127]. This suggests increasing income insecurity and the likelihood of a two-tier health service with better-resourced institutions providing the best care and conditions for staff.

The move from tax based to social insurance systems has also affected the income security of staff. The intention was to enhance efficiency and quality of provision through the introduction of detailed contracts specifying what was to be delivered and at what cost. The presumption cannot have been that any efficiency savings to be made would be at the expense of individual members of staff. Nonetheless, as the representatives of insurance organizations have introduced new payment methods based on capitation or diagnostic related groups, there is some evidence that this has undermined the position of staff (particularly non-medical staff). In Lithuania and Slovakia for example, income insecurity was felt to have increased as a result of low fee-for-service agreements and the indebtedness of sickness funds to hospitals whereas in Croatia the shift was believed to have increased income for some staff but reduced it for others (see Afford, 2001). While in Bulgaria and Slovakia physicians' associations negotiate remuneration directly with insurance companies, prompting concerns about the security of other occupational groups (see voice representation security).

The introduction of direct out-of-pocket or co-payments for pharmaceuticals and some services (in primary care, or in ambulatory clinics or for dentistry) has also been a common reform theme. It was meant to rule out informal, under-the-table payments and secure more funds for health services (particularly in countries with low tax revenues). Although the implications for staff were not a priority consideration, additional revenues and the formalising of out-of-pocket payments might have been expected to allow for greater security about income levels. Outcomes have been mixed however, the money generated from formal charges is only partially invested in pay (with some going towards clinic or hospital running costs) and staff have concerns about relying exclusively on formal payments since these are all taxed and therefore "worth less". It seems that levying charges has compromised access to health care without resolving income issues and that in many countries patients now pay both formal and informal charges (see Afford, 2001).

Privatization is a reform, which takes the concept of user charges to its ultimate extreme. It is still relatively small scale in most of CEE and CIS and tends to overlap with the establishment of small practices or clinics where self-employed physicians or dentists directly employ support staff. The evidence of its effects on income security is mixed. Wages can be higher than in the public sector, as in Georgia and the Russian Federation, less as in Latvia or on a par with the public sector as in the Czech Republic (although in more

---

[127] The *gmina* and *voivodship* both employ hospital staff with unknown consequences for pay or relative income security (Afford, 2001).

entrepreneurial organizations Czech doctors can generate significant extra income). In Slovakia, doctors in private practice earn more than if they worked for public sector while nurses are believed to earn less than their public sector counterparts (see Afford, 2001). It is unclear how the sector will develop but it is certain that there needs to be a concerted effort to ensure voice representation security if staff and their income are to be protected now and in the long run.

Reform and the focus on doctors

The effect of these various reforms on health sector pay and income security does of course vary from country to country depending on the nature of the national labour market and financial resources invested in health. It is noticeable however, that almost without exception, explicit discussion of payment mechanisms for staff (as opposed to hospitals) revolves around doctors and how best to manage their outputs and performance. This is because doctors (and on rare occasions in CEE and CIS, nurses) determine the amount of "service" given. Payment structures aim therefore to control physician actions. For example, if health system managers want to increase the number of patients seen they consider "encouraging" doctors via a piecework type system. Conversely, doctors may be paid a fixed salary to reduce the incentives for them to see and treat more patients, which will in turn keep the overall costs of drugs and procedures down. Health policy-makers see doctors' wages as being determined not by needs of the doctor, or even a vague notion of worth and skills, but very much in terms of cost containment and service outcome. The salaries of other staff receive very little attention, despite the fact that they make up the vast majority of health sector staff, because they are not regarded as motors of health service expenditure.

Typically reformers are now seeking to combine elements of salary, fee for service, and capitation in doctors' salaries in order to maximize performance. Salary is meant to provide a degree of income security and provide for routine tasks to be carried out. Fee for service creates incentives for efficiency, although it may also perversely encourage over treatment (Normand, 1998). Capitation fosters responsibility for a population as a whole and particularly for preventive measures (Rochaix, 1998). The attempt to put together different payment mechanisms in ways that reflect the interest of patients and third party payers is in marked contrast to the approach before transition (Contandriopoulos *et al.*, 1990). In centrally planned economies all staff were salaried and only in the late 1980s was any attempt made to introduce small incentive payments to encourage better practice. There is no question but that a salary provides more security than a payment structure that seeks to prompt particular behaviours. The recent reforms were designed without thinking through the impact they would have on staff and have indeed undermined income security.

Although doctors are the main targets of the reform other staff have been affected, if only as an afterthought. The creation of fund holding and capitation payments for general practitioners for example has led to doctors directly employing the nursing staff they need to deliver primary care. This puts nurses very much at a disadvantage when negotiating pay and conditions. The contracting of medical establishments by insurance companies in the Russian Federation has led to the introduction of performance related pay with significant bonuses for all outputs above a set of established norms. This in turn has given the administration enormous power in determining which staff or groups of staff are entitled to such bonuses (for details see Stepantchikova *et al.*, 2001). Again this has increased payment insecurity. Nevertheless, most nursing, administrative and support staff where they have remained in the hospital system are paid using a salary-based approach with only minor adjustments to reflect incentive schemes introduced for doctors. The neglect of these groups does little to suggest that they are valued or that their security is anyone's primary concern. It seems unlikely therefore that they will be able to muster the motivation and commitment needed to deliver more effective, efficient and responsive health care services.

Conclusions and policy recommendations

Pay in the health sector is low and staffs routinely works additional hours and additional jobs simply to earn enough to survive. It is not just the fact that pay is so poor, which causes income insecurity. It is rather a combination of circumstances. First, most staff experience or feel that they are experiencing falling real wages. Second, there are growing differences in levels of pay between different occupations in different places; and third, many staff is paid late. They have also lost in-kind benefits, which have made them more vulnerable to inflation in the cash economy, while there is no comprehensive social security system for them to fall back on.

The evidence on income security gives little cause for optimism. The policy debate gives even less. It is dominated by concern for the various dimensions of health system performance and by Western European assumptions about the role of physicians, the levers for changing professional behaviour and what motivates staff. It is hard to see why a combination of payment mechanisms designed to placate English general practitioners opposed to the national health service in 1948 should provide a gold standard for organizing family medicine in Eastern Europe, or why the fee-for-service approach that has seen German health care costs spiral should act as a model for paying doctors in Central Asia. Most worryingly there is an assumption that doctors need to be given performance related payments if they are to do their best for their patients but that nurses, cleaners and auxiliaries can continue to labour for sub-standard public sector salaries with little prospect of any significant improvement.

Corrosive reform: Failing health systems in Eastern Europe

If health system reforms are to maximize the "public good" achieved for the resources invested and if they are to encourage patient centred and responsive services they must address the needs of all the occupational groups in the sector. It is not "wrong" to adapt payment mechanisms or to introduce incentives, and too much security may foster complacency (albeit that health sector workers are a long way from this point), but unless some basic guarantees are provided then staff cannot be expected to function adequately. This means ensuring that all staff can have union representation in negotiating pay, in order to maintain some national standards for all employees. The ambivalence, even often contempt, towards trade unions displayed by some of the international agencies supporting salary structure reforms indicates that this may be a forlorn hope. However, if the health system cannot provide at least a certain level of income relative to other sectors of the economy; if it cannot sustain that income over time and in the face of inflation; and if it cannot create incentives that include all staff then the problematic and widespread custom of under-the-table payments will continue. This is undesirable from an employment perspective because it is unreliable and because it creates inappropriate inequalities between staff. (Those who have more contact with patients or more power will "earn" more than those who carry out support functions or are unassuming). It is even more undesirable from a health policy perspective since it challenges fundamentally the equal right of all patients to health care. Furthermore, if the health sector cannot address income security it is liable to see increasing numbers of trained staff take their skills and their experience and apply them in the health services of Western Europe. The following recommendations attempt to map steps that could strengthen income security and, by improving conditions for staff, improve the chances that health system objectives would be achieved.

International agencies and bilateral assistance programmes should:

- invest in programmes to support the development of civil society and to encourage compliance with tax and insurance regimes so that the countries of CEE and CIS are able to maintain adequate funding for public services;

- advocate a minimum percentage of GDP be devoted to public health expenditures;

- link investment funds to guarantees of basic payments to staff;

- recommend the formal involvement of trade unions in national pay negotiations;

- promote the indexing of the minimum wage to the average national wage;

- encourage national governments to limit differentials between occupational groups;

- sponsor a meeting to pull together all research on under-the-table payments to better understand the scale of the informal economy in health; and

- support a review of the evidence on the efficiency of performance-related pay in health.

Governments where possible should:

- commit themselves to working in partnership with unions on income, staffing and migration related issues to develop national strategies to provide income security;

- revise the minimum wage, linking it to national average earnings;

- review average pay across the health sector in light of national average earnings and realign wages accordingly;

- make a firm commitment to occupational pensions provided by the state within the health sector;

- examine differentials between occupational groups and between staff in different regions and sectors and in parallel health systems and review changing pay patterns from a gender perspective;

- scrutinize mixed-payment formulae in light of their impact on income security and the evidence on the efficiency of performance related pay;

- establish some links between the level of pay of doctors and that of auxiliary staff to ensure progression in pay across the whole health care system;

- legislate to protect the pay of staff in the private sector and in independent provider units and to outlaw late pay in any setting; and

- improve the remuneration of health sector staff, so workers are paid a decent wage on time and provided with appropriate benefits and entitlements, in order to enhance the prestige of staff and avoid under-the-table payments.

Trade unions should

- pursue through collective bargaining the best possible levels of income for staff in all occupations and in all areas;

- put pressure on the governments that have ratified ILO conventions on pay and late payments to honour the terms of those commitments;

- advocate for nationally negotiated pay frameworks that will protect staff in poorer regions and in smaller institutions and ensure pay equity;

- promote the pay claims of auxiliary staff, occupations that do not directly influence health system expenditure and those that have no direct contact with patients to ensure no group becomes marginalized or particularly insecure;

- seek to ensure that the staff in national and local health authorities with responsibilities for introducing and implementing change are included in efforts to secure decent wages and working conditions;

- monitor the pay of support staff employed by single-handed or small group practices to establish whether there is divergence from national norms;

- examine pay in the private sector and its trends relative to public sector pay;

- track differentials between occupational groups with particular reference to the pay of auxiliary or relatively unskilled staff and to ensure that any inequities based on gender are highlighted and corrected;

- negotiate with government and employers to address pensions and to resist attempts to pass responsibility for pension provision to the individual; and

- develop a communication package to allow local officials to review with members the implications of under-the-table payments for income security.

CONCLUSIONS 10

The upheaval in the economies of CEE and CIS during transition has been catastrophic for workers. Price liberalization preceded restructuring and contributed to hyperinflation. Production faltered, GDP values collapsed, and there was a break down in the collection of public revenues and taxes. Reforms destroyed much of the work-benefit regime that had guaranteed a basic level of socio-economic security for the majority of eastern Europeans. Rising unemployment, including long-term and hidden unemployment appeared for the first time in decades, yet governments singularly failed to establish the kind of comprehensive benefits systems that could have adequately protected their populations. Instead public spending was cut back, often under pressure from international agencies like the IMF and World Bank, while the informal dimension of economies burgeoned and peoples' lives become increasingly precarious.

Health workers across the region have suffered at the same time as the rest of society, although the problems they face are not identical. The nature of health and health care ensure two things, a demand for services whatever the economics of transition, and that governments and international agencies will be under pressure to see that some basic provision continues to function. Certainly the scale of job cuts and the ensuing unemployment has been markedly lower in health than in some other sectors, despite the clamour from expert advisers for action on what was portrayed as significant overstaffing. Large-scale job losses may not have materialised but labour market security has been severely compromised nevertheless. It has been diminished by the anxiety generated by the talk of cuts and by the reforms taking place, most of which the workforce believe will jeopardize jobs. Decentralization, privatization and the restructuring of primary care all involve variations on the same theme, the passing of employment contracts from the state to individual employers. Hospitals, polyclinics, dentist, diagnostic and general practices have begun to hire (and fire) staff directly, fragmenting employment, concentrating considerable power in the hands of a few senior (typically medical and often male) managers and making it more difficult for trade unions to organize and to represent workers effectively. Pressures to "modernize" and to harmonize with EU standards threaten job security. Nurses are expected to expand their roles. Whole sub-specialities are being closed down. Workers fear the future and have become less secure as a result.

They have also been beset by other material concerns. Work security has been undermined by a lack of investment in facilities and by the weakening of health and safety structures. Staff are scared to take time off work in case they lose their jobs and because they cannot afford the loss of earnings. Skill reproduction security has been undermined by the introduction of charges for training in some countries, and by the shifting of indirect costs to trainees in others. (Staff are expected to take unpaid leave to attend courses, pay for books and so on). Pay, which was never particularly high, has dropped further compared to national averages, and although doctors in some countries have won significant increases, most staff feel less able to manage and increasingly they resort to second jobs or to accepting under-the-table payments, which cannot by their nature provide real income security. Throughout this the trade union movement, which had helped to enforce safety regulations, secure access to training and protect pay, lost ground. Antipathy from neo-liberal governments, the IMF and World Bank and discouragement on the part of members eroded voice representation.

The most obvious conclusion of any analysis of the seven dimensions of health workers' security is that transition has made health sector staff significantly less secure. Reviewing their experience in the light of that of other workers does not challenge this even though there are certain features of health systems, like a guaranteed demand for their services, which have tended to protect staff a little from the changes taking place. It also seems that despite extensive upheavals and numerous reforms and reorganizations, there is a sense in which staff have managed to struggle on and to preserve much of what went before, albeit at considerable personal cost.

The reforms of health care are far from complete. It remains to be seen what the impact of further change will be on staff, or how the accession process will impinge on them. It is clear however that building a number of straightforward steps into the reform process will afford health sector workers far better protection than they have now and allow them to concentrate on improving health services performance free of the stresses and fear of job losses they experience now. These measures would reduce the likelihood of future health systems reforms being at the expense of health workers' security.

First, health policy-makers, international agencies and health care reform experts need to wake up to the implications for staff of reforming health systems. Protestations that staff and their motivation are central to the success of reforms are commonplace yet health system literature is just not adequate in the way it thinks about workers. It is exceptionally rare to find any full consideration of the impact on staff of proposed changes. Assertions that staffing levels are too high are not accompanied by attempts to measure the cost of alternative (perhaps more capital intensive) models of provision or of adding to unemployment. Neo-liberal prescriptions about minimizing government regulation do not factor in the consequences of reducing health and safety standards in a hospital setting.

Plans to change contract types and payment mechanisms (to facilitate efficiency and responsiveness) seem to ignore the evidence that insecurity undermines trust in the work place, which in turn affects performance and the service, that patients receive. If quality of care is to be an important outcome of health care reforms, then reformers need to give real consideration to how the people who provide that care are treated.

Second, planners and health economists need to go beyond their current focus on doctors and pay more attention to other occupational groups. It is no doubt true that physicians are the main drivers of expenditure in the health sector and account for all spending relating to admissions, tests and so on but doctors alone do not account for the quality of care. Training ought to address more than the shift towards family or general practice. It might, for example, develop nurses' ability to care for the elderly or the mentally ill, equip administrators with the financial management skills demanded by the changes in health sector funding or better prepare health authority staff with responsibility for managing change. By the same token, efforts to adjust job boundaries should not be premised on the idea that nurses can substitute for doctors on occasion and chiefly as a cost saving measure. Instead the possibilities of expanding the roles of a range of staff should be explored, provided of course that they are compensated for additional responsibilities. It is particularly important that the "consideration" of all occupational groups extends to pay negotiations and includes gender equity. Doctors now often have (relatively powerful) physicians' associations representing them, with direct access to third-party payers and a role in accreditation. They are also best placed to generate additional income, through private practice. If policy-makers prioritize doctors' demands over all others they run the risk of creating a health system staffed by poorly paid, poorly motivated workers who service their well rewarded medical colleagues and their patients without the desired "responsiveness" or "humanity of care".

Third, the people and organizations that make decisions about health systems need to reconsider the role of trade unions. Even though they continue to work for members' interests in difficult circumstances and with some real successes, there is no question that unions have lost some ground in terms of membership and influence. Physicians' associations have, in many countries, supplanted them in representing the sectional interests of doctors and in addressing certain issues around professional standards and insurance/reimbursement. Many governments have moved away from meaningful tripartite and social dialogue approaches. Even those agencies that recognize the importance of engaging workers' representatives are failing to include them in a strategic way. An informal survey of international health experts (so informal as not be included in the substantive analysis of this Monograph) confirmed that unions just do not figure in the thinking of many of the professionals who advise Ministries of Health. The most common response to the question "are unions present in discussions of national reforms" was (to paraphrase rather wildly), "oh we had not thought of that". Nor could anyone give an example of general unions playing a part in training, although they did report that nursing and physicians' associations and academia were all actively involved. That said there was real sympathy for the notion that unions should be part of strategic planning at the very highest level. Clearly, unions should play a crucial role in guaranteeing voice representation for a whole range of staff. They also ought to be contributing, as of course many still are, in terms of pay bargaining, regulating health and safety, testing new legislation and rethinking demarcation issues. National governments and international agencies need therefore to re-examine how they facilitate this. They need to signal who unions are to negotiate with and how these processes are to work, particularly as central government withdraws from its role as employer and in the absence of established employers' associations [128]. They also need to review how they engage with trade unions as full partners in social dialogue so that workers' representation becomes part and parcel of the way health care reforms are designed, implemented and evaluated and so that the health system can benefit from "the close interrelation between social dialogue, decent work and quality health services" (ILO, 2002b).

Fourth, more consideration should be given to the implications of European enlargement for health sector staff. A dozen CEE countries are scheduled to "accede" to the European Union over the next few years and the experience of Austrian, Finnish and Swedish accession provides very few clues as to the likely impact. EU standards and training curricula are already being adopted (even in countries that have not been given "rapid transition" status) and specialties are being restructured to meet EU norms, often without consultation with the staff affected or enough consideration of the traditions that informed national approaches. Ministries of Health and international agencies are already endeavouring to assess what accession implies for the planning of human resources and how the movement of staff and patients is likely to affect numbers entering training and the numbers who will migrate once they qualify. The problems of modulating the production of staff, supply and demand when unknown numbers will migrate westwards, and the possibility that CEE and CIS countries will end up subsidising the staff training costs of Western Europe are already on policy-makers' agendas. They must also consider how the changes being commissioned will affect existing staff and what it implies for their future careers. This is particularly important if, as is likely, younger staff, trained to new standards and criteria are targeted for recruitment by richer EU Member States, leaving "behind" an experienced workforce but one with a relatively narrow skill and age profile.

Fifth, more research is needed to understand what is actually happening to workers. It is already clear from the ILO/PSI survey and from informal

---

[128] For practical guidance for policy-makers implementing public service and health sector reforms see WHO (2002a).

responses to questions posed to PSI affiliates that there is a vast gap between what workers are entitled to on paper and what happens in practice. It seems that many staff routinely work overtime without pay because of a mixture of coercion and conviction. Some feel that they cannot say no to employers or to double shifts, others cover for colleagues who are ill, most are motivated by "altruism", "vocation" or "responsibility" and work additional, unpaid hours rather than leave patients without adequate support. Their extra shifts do not appear in hospital statistics. The almost region wide fall in absenteeism is another area where official figures do not capture the reality. Some of the drop can be attributed to changes in custom and practice. (Before transition, it was normal for staff in some countries to "use up" their sick leave entitlement, but this has changed as employment insecurity has increased.) Some is due to the new phenomenon of "presenteeism". (Sick pay is so much lower than the daily wage and workers are so afraid of losing their jobs that staff who are sick still go to work.) Again the data do not uncover what is actually happening. There are also glaring gaps in knowledge, which can only be addressed by further research. The parallel health services are a case in point. It is unclear how many health workers are employed by other Ministries or by enterprises, how they are represented and what the implications of further health sector reform will be for them. Similarly, not enough is known about gender and security; the contracting out of services; or health care workers in rural areas; or the role of under-the-table payments in household income; or of the extent to which the minimum wage levels impact on health sector pay; or exactly why reports of accidents and injuries have fallen so steeply. Research is needed if policy-making is going to become increasingly evidence-based and reflect the real stresses that workers face. There is also evidence and analysis from other European countries, and other regions, that could usefully be made available to CEE and CIS policy-makers, and which would allow them to incorporate an understanding of the consequences of decisions tested elsewhere into their own policy formulation.

Finally, the health systems literature suggests that any one of a number of models of tax-based or social health insurance funding can provide reasonably equitable health care coverage and that it is legitimate for countries to choose between them depending on context and preference. It also suggests that shifting from one model to another cannot succeed in the face of immense resource scarcity and wholesale economic disruption. The evidence from the region bears this out. It is clear that many of the health system reforms of the last 12 years have created enormous socio-economic insecurity. This was absolutely not their intention nor was it a direct consequence (in most cases) of the reform model chosen. It was rather that governments engaged in root and branch reorganization of health care when there were neither the resources nor the technical wherewithal to accomplish the reforms necessary. This is not to argue that health systems could have remained untouched by the changes of transition. It is however to suggest that the scale of reforms undertaken and the ideological commitment to change for change sake were ill advised. The reforms that perhaps 'should not have been attempted' have clearly, if inadvertently damaged the people who work in the health sector. It is important therefore that governments and their advisers learn the lessons of a decade of transition and carry out the analysis that is needed to ensure that future reforms are feasible, manageable and sustainable and are not achieved at the expense of workers' security.

Health, unlike other "commodities" is permanently "in demand". The health services of CEE and CIS will always employ huge numbers of staff even though the exact size of the sector may vary. If they are not to create a vast, permanent working poor or to perpetuate insecure employment then policy-makers must create an opportunity to address the needs of health workers. Talking to them and to their representatives would not be a bad starting point.

The following recommendations are intended to identify areas for action that cut across the seven dimensions of socio-economic security and address some of the challenges facing health sector staff in the round. They are intended not for any one group but to suggest areas where all health sector stakeholders can work together to create health services that promote the health and well-being of staff and users alike.

International agencies and bilateral assistance programmes, governments, trade unions and associations should:

- explicitly recognize that the sheer scale of the health sector as an employer gives it very real macro-economic significance and reflect this in their approach to the sector;

- state clearly and unequivocally that the treatment of health sector workers, their socio-economic security, in all its dimensions, and their well-being are important in and of themselves and because they have a direct impact on the health sector's ability to deliver high quality, efficient and responsive care;

- agree that social dialogue and the inclusion of trade unions and associations, local health authorities, government, third-party payers and employers as full partners in discussions at all appropriate planning and decision-making levels (together with appropriate involvement of user-organizations and other stakeholders) is central to the strategic development of the health care system nationally and locally (ILO, 2002b);

- review the employment impact of all proposed reforms as they are developed and implemented, including any suggested changes in contract type;

- develop and communicate clearly a 'road map' of reforms so that workers can get a sense of the scale of the intended change and their place in it;

- address national and local investment priorities so that adequate infrastructure and health and safety are guaranteed before high technology is acquired and so that male and female workers benefit from the investments made;

- include the staff of parallel health services and those working in decentralized settings, small or independent practices and the private sector in all policy deliberations, ensuring that equity and their socio-economic security are considered fully;

- establish a national framework for pay and conditions that protects against undue regional inequality or inappropriate or gender based differentials, and allows for the review of any proposed changes in payment formula in light of their impact on income security and equity;

- endeavour to secure adequate pay, pensions and benefits (and payment on time), for all occupational groups in all health service settings and with the opportunity to increase wages appropriately over time, including lobbying to secure a sufficient share of GDP for health to achieve this;

- engage in joint action to address the problems in collecting taxes and insurance contributions and the practice of under-the-table payments, which diminish the funds available to pay for the health sector;

- work to agree a legislative framework which will enshrine the existing protection that workers have and extend that protection to include the entitlement to belong to a trade union, to be consulted about job changes and to have all rights protected in the event that their employment contract is transferred to another employer (whether that be a decentralized public sector body or a private sector contractor);

- provide effective (useable) training and retraining without charge (direct or indirect) for all staff including managers and most particularly for those whose jobs are affected by changing standards, ensuring that they are fully consulted and that retraining allows them to take on new roles and functions and pursue alternative development paths, consistent with the reforms;

- ensure that the institutions are accredited, that accreditation includes reference to training provision, health and safety and the approach to staff socio-economic security and that all social partners, including trade unions, are involved in the accreditation process;

- monitor the consequences of EU enlargement, not only in terms of the movement of staff and the loss of qualified and dynamic personnel, but also as it affects planning of staff production, job boundaries, the disappearance of culturally appropriate specialities, and the morale of remaining staff;

- research into the reality of the experience of health systems staff addressing late pay, administrative leave, reliance on under-the-table benefits, absenteeism, health and safety, violence and gender issues and disseminate data and case-studies that serve to illuminate the insecurity of staff; and

- create networks and channels of communications between partners for social dialogue, including between trade unions and associations, and with international counterparts to promote the sharing of views, better understanding of concepts and terminology, training and the transfer of experience and learning between actors, regions and countries.

POSTCRIPTS
— LATEST DEVELOPMENTS IMPACTING
ON HEALTH AND SOCIAL SERVICES

The Czech Republic

On 1 January 2003, the next stage of the reform of public administration in the Czech Republic came into force. The objective was to get the public administration and services closer to the citizens, with the role of the state further decentralised and de-concentrated. The objective, however, has not been reached successfully. Many powers of the state were supposed to be taken over by newly constructed self-governing regions. Unfortunately, various areas within the public services had not been prepared for the changes. In transferring powers from the state to regional and local governments, the central government underestimated the need to first solve issues related to the rights of those establishing, or founding, public services, and to set standards for access and quality of services, as well as to prepare sufficient public funding. The funds that have been transferred to the new, independent self-governing units are insufficient to enable the public services to carry out their new responsibilities.

The decision-making process concerning social services has become more distant for the citizens in the Czech Republic, having moved from the district to the regional level. Local communities, not having been granted sufficient funding from the state, refused to take over the duties of running such services that had been provided previously by state-run institutions (including both non-resident and long-term institutional social services). Consequently, these too were transferred to the regional level. The regions are not obliged to observe any provisions concerning accessibility to services. Presently, changes in the tax system are under consideration to get a larger part of the tax base channelled directly to the regions. However, it is not yet clear when the new system should come into force and with what consequences.

A new law on social services is being prepared at present. A representative of our trade union is a member of the working group of the Ministry of Labour and Social Affairs. In the area of social services, there is no organisation of employers, which could function as a social partner, with whom it would be possible to bargain collectively.

The newly established regions have taken over the former role of the state in establishing and running health care institutions. They have taken over establishing regional emergency services and hospitals comprising about two thirds of hospital beds in the whole country. This happened at the time when hospitals have a debt of 2.5 milliard Czech Krowns a year because of the demonstrated non-profitability of the hospital sector. The regions refuse to take over the indebted hospitals and want to change the present status of the hospitals to joint-stock companies with 100 per cent ownership of the region. These joint-stock companies would control the immovable property of the region. Trade unions are concerned that the relations and rules are becoming so complicated that the continuity of labour relations and employment and working conditions might be endangered, as well as the salaries of the workers. If the employees became workers of a commercial institution, they would lose their right to the state-guaranteed pay based on established pay scales. No nationwide or even regional collective agreement has been concluded in the sector, and because of obstruction by the employers, negotiations are only in an infant working stage, which serves to exacerbate these difficulties.

The Trade Union of the Health Service and Social Care of the Czech Republic has been preparing information about the essential parts of establishment documents and statutes of business companies. This information is to be used by the workers and their trade union organisations. The union has also started negotiations with all 14 regional governments about the practical implementation outlined in these documents.

Ukraine: Wage payment in health sector

The situation in the health sector and socio-economic protection of health workers in Ukraine is extremely poor due to very limited financing. This has resulted in a level of pay that is lower than the officially recognized subsistence minimum for the working population and therefore health workers face great difficulty in meeting their basic needs. (The average wage of health workers is UAH 235, USD 44, and the subsistence minimum of able-bodied population is UAH 365, USD 68.)

Article 77, of the Grounds of Health Protection Legislation, is not being observed in terms of the obligation to increase the official salary in the health sector to the same level as the average wage in industry including the provision of privileges provided for by the legislation.

The lack of real mechanisms to ensure legal and socio-economic security has led to a decline in the public recognition of health workers', therefore lowering of their status and devaluing their work. This in turn undermines the constitutional right of Ukrainian citizens to be provided with adequate health care.

The Government ignored the demand, signed by over 660'000 health workers, to find a solution to the socio-economic problems of the sector. This resulted in a collective labour dispute. The National Conciliation and Mediation Service registered the collective labour dispute between the Health Workers' Union and the Ministry of Health Protection of Ukraine (i.e. the Government) by its decree of 29 December 2001, however this dispute has not been settled so far.

The major demand was for an improvement in the existing socio-economic working conditions for health workers according to the current legislation. To create conditions for ensuring decent wages for health workers, who work round-the-clock, often in hazardous health conditions, and taking responsibility for patients.

On the initiative of the health workers' union the Cabinet of Ministers of Ukraine issued a Decree # 1298 of 30 August 2002 on Workers' Wage Payment based on a single tariff scale of ranks and coefficients for workers of budget sector institutions, including health workers, that should have come in force on 1 January 2003. But by the Decree of the Cabinet of Ministers of Ukraine of 25 December 2002 # 1270 on Amendments to the Decree of the Cabinet of Ministers of Ukraine of 30 August 2002 # 1298 its effect was delayed until the second quarter of 2003. According to the trade union's data this term is not final.

From the health union's point of view the Ministry of Labour and Social Policy is in the process of setting the first rank tariff according to the new single tariff scale at a rate which is below the minimum wage without consulting the trade union's and contrary to the ILO Convention 98 and to the national legislation.

The main issue from the trade union perspective is that with the introduction of the single tariff scale the rate of the health worker's salary of the first tariff rank should not be lower than the minimum wage.

REFERENCES [129]

Afford C. 2001. Failing health systems: Failing health care workers in Eastern Europe (Geneva, ILO).

Brusati, L. *et al*. 2002. "Health care systems in transition: Belarus", in European Observatory on Health Care Systems (Copenhagen, in press).

Busse R. *et al*. 2000. "Health care systems in transition: Czech Republic", European Observatory on Health Care Systems (Copenhagen).

Cerniauskas, G. *et al*. 2000. "Health care systems in transition: Lithuania", in European Observatory on Health Care Systems (Copenhagen).

Chenet, L. *et al*. 1996. "Changing life expectancy in Central Europe: Is There a Single Reason?," in Journal of Public Health Medicine, p. 18.

Chetvernina *et al*. 1997. "Establishment of a system of unemployment insurance in Russia" in G. Standing The Folly of Social Safety Nets: Why Basic Income is Needed in Eastern Europe, p. 8.

Contandriopoulos A.P. *et al*. 1990. "Systèmes de soins et modalités de remunération. Sociologie du travail 1", in R. Saltman and J. Figueras European Health Care Reform, Analysis of Current Strategies (Copenghagen, WHO Regional Publications, European Series), No. 72.

Department of Statistics of Lithuania. 1999. Demographic Yearbook, 1998 (Vilnius).

Domagala, A *et al*. 2000. Public Service Reforms and Their Impact on Health Sector Personnel: Case Studies on Cameroon, Colombia, Jordan, Philippines, Poland and Uganda (Geneva, ILO), pp. 169–207

Dunford, M and Smith, A. 2000. "Catching up or falling behind? Economic performance and regional trajectories in the "new" Europe", in Economic Geography 76 (2).

---

[129] This Reference lists the sources used for this Monograph and includes additional references that were integral to the reports that fed into it, namely Afford, 2001; Stepantchikova *et al.*, 2001 and ILO, 2001.

Corrosive reform: Failing health systems in Eastern Europe

Economist Intelligence Unit (EIU). 2001. Business Environment Scores and Ranks (London), August.

Elliot, R. 1998. "Labour economics: A comparative analysis (London; McGraw Hill 1991)", cited in Critical Challenges for Health Care Reform in Europe, World Health Organization (Buckingham, Open University Press).

EU PHARE. 1996). Romania Report. www.lshtm.ac

Fashoyin, T. 2002. The contribution of social dialogue to economic and social development in Zambia, ILO InFocus Programme on Strengthening Social Dialogue Working Paper and referred to in the Draft Report to the Joint Meeting on the Social Dialogue in Health Services: Institutions, Capacity and Effectivenes, pp. 70–75.

Gamkrelidze, A. *et al.* 2002. "Health care systems in transition: Georgia", in European Observatory on Health Care Systems (Copenhagen).

General Health Insurance Company of the Czech Republic. 2000. Annual Report for 2000 (Prague, General Health Insurance Company of the Czech Republic).

German Foundation for International Development (DSE). 2000. Public Service Reforms and Their Impact on Health Sector Personnel (DSE, Berlin).

Hall, D. 1998. Cited in Workshop on Employment and Labour Practices in Health Care in Central and Eastern Europe, Joint Report by the International Labour Organization/Public Services International (Geneva, ILO), p. 22.

Healy, J. and Humphries, C. 1997. Health Care Personnel in Central and Eastern Europe (Geneva, ILO Sectoral Working Paper).

Hovhannisyan, S. *et al.* 2001. "Health care systems in transition: Armenia", in European Observatory on Health Care Systems (Copenhagen).

Hunter, D. 1998. Cited in Workshop on Employment and Labour Practices in Health Care in Central and Eastern Europe, Joint Report by the International Labour Organization/Public Services International (Geneva, ILO).

Institute of Health Information. 2000. Czech Health Statistics Yearbook 1999 (Prague, Institute of Health Information).

International Labour Organization (ILO). 1992. Note on the proceedings, Standing Technical Committee for Health and Medical Services, First Session, (Geneva, ILO)

_____. 1997. ILO Yearbook of Statistics (Geneva, ILO).

_____. 1998. ILO/PSI Workshop on Employment and Labour Practices in Health Care in Central and Eastern Europe, Prague 1997 (Geneva, ILO).

_____. 1999. ILO InFocus Programme on Socio-Economic Security — A Medium-Term Work Plan (Geneva, ILO).

_____. 2000. Current International Recommendations on Labour Statistics (Geneva, ILO), pp. 20–23.

_____. 2000a. Employment and Working Conditions in the Health Sector of Central Asian countries, Report for the International Labour Office and Public Services International (Geneva, ILO).

_____. 2001. Health Care in Central and Eastern Europe: Reform, Privatization and Employment in Four countries, Draft Report to the ILO InFocus Programme on Socio-Economic Security and Public Services International (Geneva, ILO).

_____. 2002. ILO/ICN/WHO/PSI Framework Guidelines for Addressing Workplace Violence in the Health Sector, Joint Programme on Workplace Violence in the Health Sector (Geneva, ILO).

_____. 2002a. Draft Report of the Joint Meeting on Social Dialogue in the Health Services: Institutions, Capacity and Effectiveness, October (Geneva, ILO).

_____. 2002b. Conclusions on Strengthening Social Dialogue in the Health Services: A Framework for Practical Guidance, Joint Meeting on Social Dialogue in the Health Services: Institutions, Capacity and Effectiveness, Geneva October (Geneva, ILO).

Kanavos, P. and McKee, M. 1998. "Macroeconomic constraints and health challenges facing European health systems", in R. Saltman et. al. Critical Challenges for Health Care Reform in Europe, World Health Organization (Buckingham, Open University Press).

Karaskevica, J. et al. 2001. "Health care systems in transition: Latvia", in European Observatory on Health Care Systems (Copenhagen).

Karski, J.B. et al. 1999. "Health care systems in transition: Poland", in European Observatory on Health Care Systems (Copenhagen).

Koulaksuzov and Todorova. 2002. "Health care systems in transition: Bulgaria", in European Observatory on Health Care Systems (Copenhagen, in press).

Macroeconomic Commission for Health. 2002. www.who.int

MacLehose L. *et al.* 2000. "Health care systems in transition: The Republic of Moldova", in European Observatory on Health Care Systems (Copenhagen, in press).

McKee, M and Healy, J. (eds). 2002. Hospitals in a Changing Europe (Buckingham and Philadelphia, Open University Press).

Marree, J. and Groenewegen, P. P. 1997. Back to Bismark: Eastern European Health Care in Transition (Avebury).

Ministry of Health. (Lithuania). The Lithuanian Health Programme (Republic of Lithuania).

National Training Fund. 2000. Human Resources in the Czech Republic 1999 (Prague, Institute for Information on Education).

Normand, C. 1998. Cited in Workshop on Employment and Labour Practices in Health Care in Central and Eastern Europe, Joint Report by the International Labour Organization/Public Services International (Geneva, ILO).

Parliamentary Hearings. 2000. Socio-Economic Status of Health Care Workers (Moscow), April 12-13.

Rainnie, A. *et. al* 2002. "Employment and work restructuring in transition," in Rainnie et. al, Work, Employment and Transition: Restructuring Livelihoods in Post-Communism (Routledge, London).

Rochaix, L. 1998. "Performance-tied payment systems for physicians", in R. Saltman et. al Critical Challenges for Health Care Reform in Europe, World Health Organization (Open University Press, Buckingham).

Russian Federation Government Report. 1992. On Health Care (Moscow).

_____. 1999. On the State of Health of the Population of the Russian Federation (Moscow).

_____. 2000. On the State of Health of the Population of the Russian Federation (Moscow).

Russian Federation Ministry of Health Care. 1996. The Health of the Population of Russia and the Activity of Health Care Establishments (Moscow).

_____. 2000. The health of the population of Russia and the activity of health care establishments (Moscow).

_____. 2001a. Information letter about the state of occupational incidence among health care workers (Moscow, Federal Centre of Governmental Sanitary and Epidemiological Supervision).

_____. 2001b. On the process of realization of the health care and medical science development concept, the tasks for the years of 2001-2005 and for the period till the year of 2010 (Moscow).

Saltman, R. and Figueras, J. 1997. European health care reform: Analysis of current strategies (Copenghagen, WHO Regional Publications, European Series), No 72.

Sargaldakova, A. *et al.* 2000. "Health care systems in transition: Kyrgyzstan", in European Observatory on Health Care Systems (Copenhagen).

Scheil-Adlung, X. 2001. Building social security: The challenge of privatization (International Social Security Series, Transaction Publishers, New Brunswick).

Schlanger, J. 2000. "Health care in the Czech Republic 1998-2000", in A Trade Union View (Prague).

Scrivens, E. 1997. Accreditation: Protecting the professional or the consumer (Buckingham, Open University Press).

Standing, G. 1996. "Social protection in Central and Eastern Europe: A tale of slipping anchors and torn safety nets," in G. Esping-Andersen (ed.), Welfare States in Transition: National Adaptations in Global Economies (Sage Publications, London).

_____. 1997. "The folly of social safety nets: Why basic income is needed in Eastern Europe," in Social Research (New York, The Graduate Faculty), Vol 64, No.4.

_____. 2002. "The babble of euphemisms: Re-embedding social protection in 'transformed' labour markets," in A. Rainnie et. al.Work, Employment and Transition: Restructuring Livelihoods in Post-Communism (Routledge, London).

Stepanchikova, N. *et al.* 2001. Socio-economic status of health care workers in the Russian Federation (Geneva, ILO).

Tomev, L et al. Forthcoming. Workplace violence in the health sector - Country Case Study: Bulgaria, Joint Programme on Workplace Violence in the Health Sector; forthcoming working paper, (Geneva, ILO)

Trade Links. 2000. Czech Republic Labour Code (Prague, Trade Links).

Thirkell, J and Vickerstaff, S. 2002. "Trade unions and the politics of transformation in Central and Eastern Europe", in A. Rainnie et al. Work, Employment and Transition: Restructuring Livelihoods in Post-communism (Routledge, London).

Tragakes, E. *et al.* 2002. "Health care systems in transition: Russia", in European Observatory on Health Care Systems (Copenhagen, in press).

United Nations (UN). 2000. Human Development Report, 2000, Romania.

Vladescu, C. *et. al.* 2000. "Health care systems in transition: Romania", in European Observatory on Health Care Systems (Copenhagen).

Vulic, S. *et al.* 1999. "Health care systems in transition: Croatia", in European Observatory on Health Care Systems (Copenhagen).

World Bank. 2000. Memorandum of the President of the International Bank for Reconstruction and Development of the International Finance Corporation to the Executive Directors on a Country Assistance Strategy for Ukraine (Washington), Report No. 20723-UA, August.

_____. 2001. Country Report Moldova. www.worldbank.org

World Health Organization (WHO). 1999. World Health Report, 1999. Databases (Copenhagen).

_____. 2000c. Highlights on Health in Ukraine.

_____. 2001a. WHO/ILO/ICN/PSI Public service reforms and their impact on health sector personnel: Critical questions: A Tool for Action (Geneva, WHO, ILO, ICN, PSI)

_____. 2001b. The World Health Report 2000. Health systems: Improving performance (Geneva).

_____. 2002a. Report of the Commission on Macroeconomics and Health. Macroeconomics and Health: Investing in Health for Economic Development (www3.whoint/whosis/cmh/cmhreport).

_____. 2002b. World Health Organization Regional Office for Europe, Health for All.

Zapoliskiene, S. 2001. The survey of the Lithuanian economy (Vilnius, Ministry of Economy, Statistics Department of Lithuania), May.

INDEX

Note: Page numbers in **bold** refer to major text sections, those in *italics* to tables and figures.

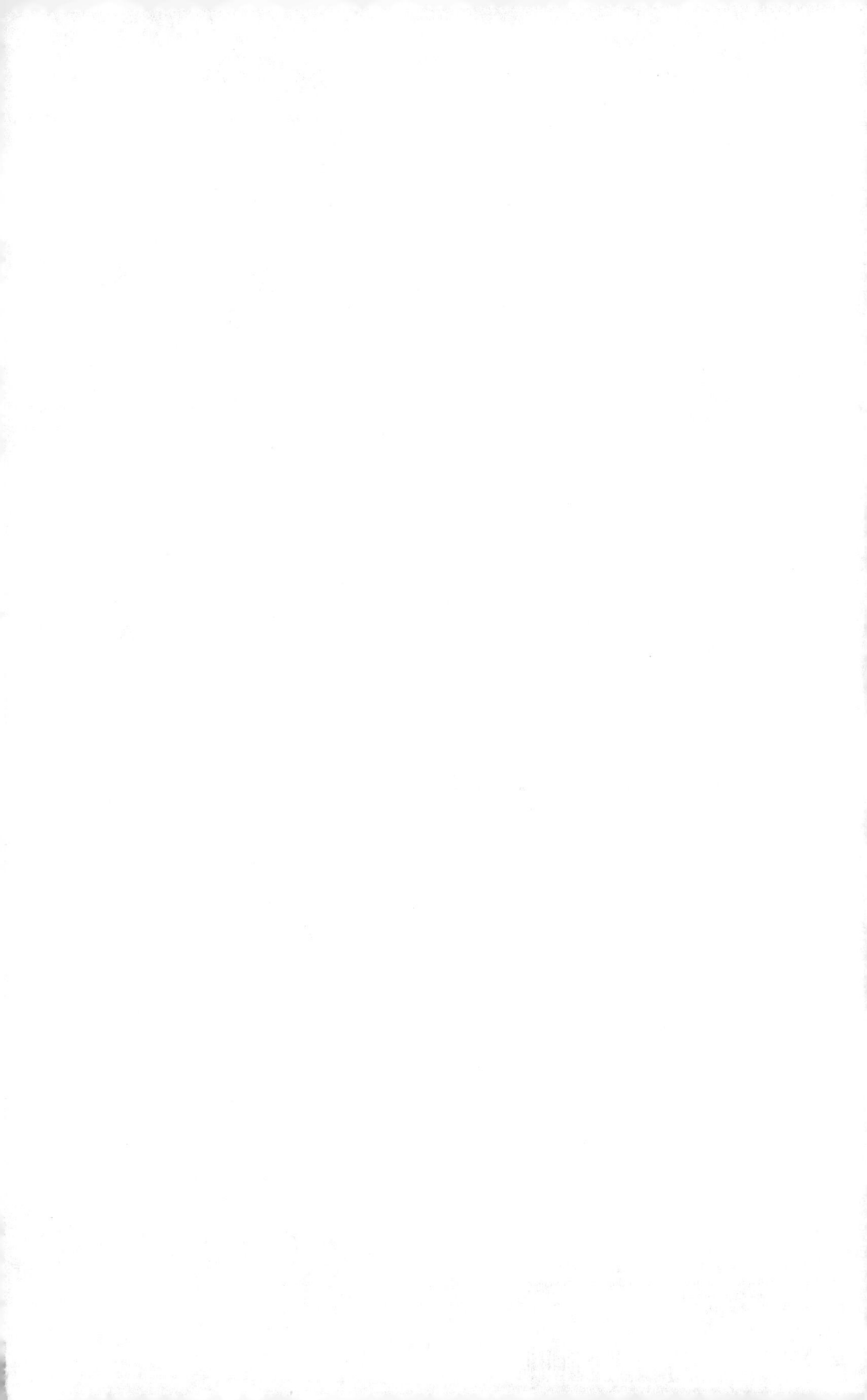

www.ingramcontent.com/pod-product-compliance
Lightning Source LLC
Chambersburg PA
CBHW070401200326
41518CB00011B/2015